Gut Crisis

HOW DIET, PROBIOTICS, AND
FRIENDLY BACTERIA HELP YOU
**LOSE WEIGHT AND HEAL
YOUR BODY AND MIND**

Robert Keith Wallace, PhD
and Samantha Wallace

Dharma Publications

Also by
Dr. Robert Keith Wallace and
Samantha Wallace

An Introduction to Transcendental Meditation
Improve Your Brain Functioning, Create Ideal Health, and
Gain Enlightenment Naturally, Easily, Effortlessly

Transcendental Meditation
A Scientist's Journey to Happiness, Health, and Peace

The Neurophysiology of Enlightenment
How the Transcendental Meditation and TM-Sidhi Program
Transform the Functioning of the Human Body

Maharishi Ayurveda and Vedic Technology
Creating Ideal Health for the Individual and World

Dharma Parenting
Understand your Child's Brilliant Brain for Greater
Happiness, Health, Success, and Fulfillment
(co-authored with Fred Travis)

Quantum Golf
The Path to Golf Mastery
(co-authored with Kjell Enhager)

To our children Eden, Ted, Gareth, and Lila,
and their dear families

ISBN 978-0-9990558-2-3

Library of Congress Control Number: 2017908401

DharmaPublications.com

Dharma Publications, Fairfield, IA

"All disease begins in the gut."

— Hippocrates

Contents

PART 4: Doc Gut's Favorite Books

PART 5: Past and Future

PART 6: What You Can Do

Authors' Note

A major health crisis is taking place around the world in the form of epidemics of such conditions as obesity, diabetes, and autoimmune disease. The root cause of these and many other diseases can all be traced back to the gut. Medical science is beginning to understand what the ancients have known for centuries: an imbalanced gut leads to disease. It begins with a break in the gut wall, followed by a local inflammatory response. This leads to a chronic state of inflammation, which is the source of disorders ranging from heart disease to Alzheimer's.

A personal journey to gut health began with an interest in gut bacteria and culminated with a startling revelation about our own health. *Gut Crisis* includes practical issues that affect everyone's health:

- What disorders are caused by an imbalanced state of gut bacteria?

- How do gut bacteria affect your cravings and emotions?

- What are the effects of probiotics?

- What is your personal Gut/Brain Nature?

- What can you do to heal your gut?

Each chapter of the book is organized in the form of a blog with a Q&A comment section that introduces three characters with different points of view: Doc Gut, Ms. Natural, and H Bomb.

Gut Crisis cuts through the volume of conflicting gut information on the Internet to help you make the best possible choices for your health and the health of your loved ones.

Introduction

I have spent much of my life lecturing at universities and scientific institutes around the world, and my typical talk is about enlightenment and its scientific verification. Last night, however, I spoke to several hundred people about the human gut and my subject went from the sublime to the revolting.

I began by pointing out that everyone seems to have some instinctive understanding that there is something powerful and fundamental about the gut. Perhaps that's why we use expressions like "trust your gut," "from the gut," "gut instincts," and "gut feelings." A brave person has "a lot of guts," while a weak person might be disparaged as "gutless."

I decided to ease into specifics of the gut by beginning with a subject of popular interest, probiotics. Probiotics are living bacteria that enter our gut and merge with other microorganisms living there, and every health store stocks them, either in the form of a pill or a drink. The "microbiome" is a name scientists use to describe all of the microorganisms in or on us, including their vast amount of genetic material. In our gut alone, we have 30 to 40 trillion bacteria cells—about the same number as all of the other cells in our body.

Why are these tiny organisms important? Bacteria can communicate with every part of our body, especially with our brain. Gut bacteria are essential to our physical and mental well-being, to the point of determining how happy or sad we are.

Gut research is not a passing health fad. The National Institutes of Health lists almost 1000 human clinical trials presently exploring the effectiveness of probiotics to treat a wide variety of diseases.

The zinger in last night's lecture was that one of the most powerful discoveries in gut research is the success of fecal transplant, a procedure in which a doctor inserts stool or "poop" from a healthy donor into the lower gut of a sick person. Before I finished this sentence, I could see looks of disgust and discomfort pass over the faces of my audience.

I tried to soften their shock by pointing out that top medical researchers around the world have found that fecal transplant is the very best treatment for an often fatal infection caused by the bacteria *Clostridium difficile*. Affecting half a million people in the United States, this disease results in severe bouts of reoccurring diarrhea and accounts for 15,000 deaths each year.

Fecal transplant is 90% effective in curing *C. difficile*. There are currently over 100 human clinical trials on the use of fecal transplant for this and other diseases. And these trials are conducted to the gold standard of modern research, often costing millions of dollars.

In the past, our focus was primarily on "bad" bacteria, which happen to be small in number compared to "good" bacteria.

Historically, most gut bacteria have been difficult to study because they don't consume oxygen and can't be easily grown in cultures. It is the development of new technologies, particularly gene sequencing, which has recently made it possible to study over 1000 different bacterial organisms. This enormous variety of bacteria live in the lower portion of our digestive tract and affect everything from anxiety to weight gain to aging.

In 1907, Nobel Prize Laureate Ilya Ilyich Mechnikov promoted probiotics in the form of Bulgarian yogurt as a means of maintaining better health and slowing the aging process. No one took him seriously at the time. Today, however, new articles are constantly being published, revealing how the state of our gut bacteria affects heart disease, diabetes, Alzheimer's, Parkinson's, multiple sclerosis, Crohn's, autism, and many other conditions.

I concluded my talk, stating that we are at the beginning of the next great revolution in modern medicine—a revolution, which will connect advanced technologies with ancient health practices and lay bare the mysteries that surround the diseases plaguing humankind.

Editorial note: We have chosen to use the term "bacteria" to mean both a single bacterium and a group of bacteria. The Latin names of bacteria are in italics, and the first word is often abbreviated. *Clostridium difficile*, for example, may be referred to as *C. difficile*.

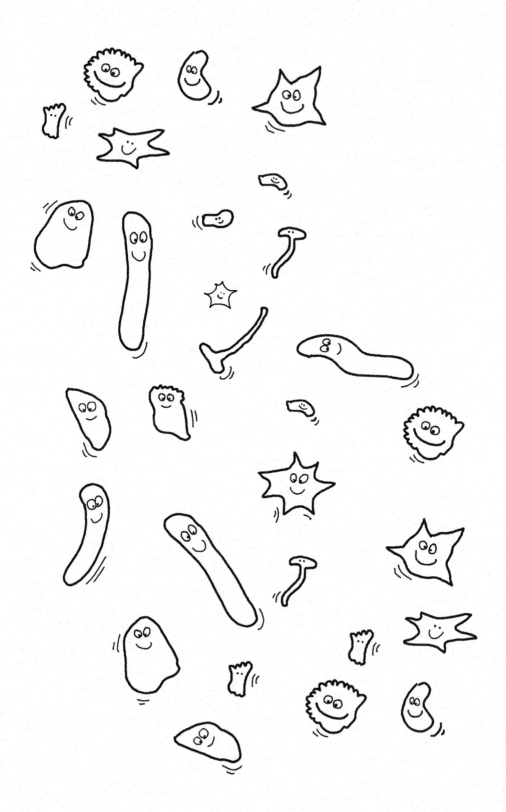

PART I

OUR HIDDEN ORGAN

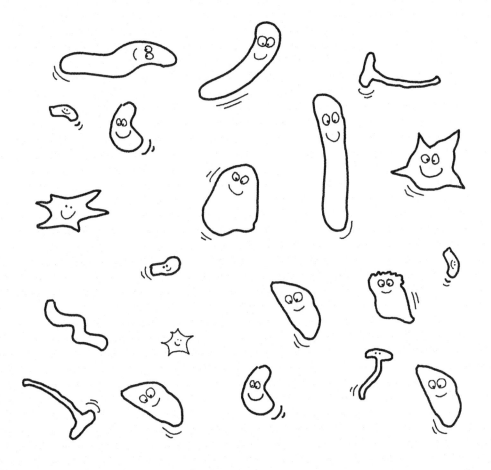

CHAPTER 1

Table Talk

At a dinner party, the woman sitting beside me asked what I considered to be "the most exciting new area of medical research."

Now, it's one thing to lecture about the inner workings of the body; it's another to discuss it at the dinner table. But she had told me earlier that she was unhappy about being overweight and I wanted to help her.

"Fecal transplant and gut bacteria!" I exclaimed, probably the last thing she was expecting me to say.

I could have politely avoided the topic, but this would suggest that I possess a degree of self-control over my scientific enthusiasm. I don't. Could I have switched to a more polite topic? Easily. The answer I gave was based on an amazing experiment in which fecal transplant dramatically reduced obesity.

This weight reduction study had been unique for two reasons: First, it involved both humans and animals. Second, it was a success. Fecal samples were taken from two adult human twins, identical in all respects except that one of them was obese, while the other was lean. One twin had become fat and the other thin.

When the fecal sample from the fat twin was transplanted into a normal size mouse, the mouse became fat. And when a sample was taken from the thin twin and transplanted into another normal size mouse, that mouse became thin. The question that naturally arose from this research is: Can human obesity be remedied by transplanting stool from thin people into fat people?

At this point, the answer is: Nobody knows. But as unpleasant as the procedure may at first seem, if these experiments work consistently well on humans, it will be an epic breakthrough in the field of weight management. Much of the developed world is in the midst of an obesity epidemic. Obesity is a major health risk factor in the development of heart disease and diabetes. No one knows whether the epidemic is due to sugar and processed food, or to the increase in stress in our lives, but it's happening everywhere, and our children are getting fatter and fatter. One fact is clear when we watch 600-pound individuals on reality TV: Obesity is all around us and it's not going away easily.

Before I could tell my dinner partner about the experiment with the twins, I had to explain the basics of fecal transplant. I began by telling her about the astounding success of fecal transplant in a study reported in the *New England Journal of Medicine*. The fecal transplant proved so much more effective and less expensive than a treatment using a strong antibiotic that the hospital deemed it unethical to continue giving the antibiotic to the patients, and stopped the study.

I want you to know that I did show some social restraint by keeping my mouth shut and not sharing an even more shocking procedure in which researchers took fecal transplant to the next level, "Poop in a Pill." Yes, you read it right. Children infected with *C. difficile* were given an oral-fecal transplant with great success. However, the technique has recently come into question. A commercial company, Seres Therapeutics, received $120 million in funding from Nestlé to create a cocktail of select highly purified gut microbes from the poop of healthy donors and put it into an oral pill form to treat *C. difficile* patients. Though initial findings were promising, later trials were unsuccessful and news of this failed trial caused Seres stock to plummet 78%. Nevertheless, the research continues.

Numerous fecal transplant clinical trials are being conducted on other conditions, including ulcerative colitis and obesity. These studies are in a preliminary stage, and there are many questions that must still be answered. How, for example, do researchers know who is the best fecal donor candidate? Should it be a relative, a best friend, or a healthy stranger? What is the best way to obtain a sample and store it? What was it that went wrong when researchers tried to purify the stool sample and put it into pill form? Can fecal transplant cure other diseases?

I spared my dinner guest this part of the discussion, and I hope that she will forgive me for ruining her appetite by bringing up this extremely promising, yet conversationally awkward, subject.

Gut Rap Q & A:

H Bomb: I like your blog, but whatta load of crap! Are you trying to tell us that squirting someone's poop into a fat guy will make him skinny?

Doc Gut: Right now, the main clinical use of fecal transplant is to cure the dangerous *C. difficile* infection. It is usually only given after the most powerful antibiotic drugs have failed. As I pointed out, fecal transplant is over 90% effective and has been a lifesaver for many people. *C. difficile* infection is a very serious problem. In some areas of the US, it is considered to be the number one hospital infection, even more prevalent and dangerous than MRSA (methicillin-resistant *Staphylococcus aureus*).

H Bomb: I have another question. Why do dogs eat poop?

Doc Gut: The easiest answer is that it allows them to consume undigested nutrients in the poop. The technical name for animals eating poop is coprophagia. And about 30% of both human and dog poop consists of gut bacteria, so it is also kind of an oral fecal transplant that allows animals to reseed their gut bacteria. I googled the words "animals eat poop" and the first thing that came up was a quote from a *National Geographic* article: "Dung beetles, rabbits, chimps, and domestic dogs are among animals that are members of the dung diners' club."

H Bomb: You're making me sick.

Ms. Natural: Aren't there records in early Traditional Chinese Medicine of patients ingesting a fecal preparation?

Doc Gut: Yes, I have heard of that.

H Bomb: Yeah, well, you'll never catch me doing it!

Ms. Natural: I heard there might someday be medical boutiques that offer selections of the healthiest, finest stool samples, and people could choose exactly the one they wanted.

H Bomb: What if they put in the wrong poop?

Doc Gut: It's standard practice for healthy family relatives to be donors and there's one well-cited case study in which a woman with *C. difficile* used her daughter as a donor for her fecal transplant. The woman was cured of her infection, but she later became obese, without altering her diet. The researchers noted that her daughter had been healthy with a normal weight at the time they took the sample, but later gained 30 pounds. To account for this, it was suggested that the mother gained weight after the procedure because the transplant included certain bacteria that promoted obesity.

H Bomb: Sounds like a messed-up science experiment.

Doc Gut: The researchers from the study recommended that greater care be taken in selecting healthy donors. If you want to look up this type of study, be sure to use the technical name for the procedure, fecal microbiome transplant or FMT.

H Bomb: Why don't they forget about poop transplant and poop pills, and stick to oral probiotics?

Doc Gut: Good question. Oral probiotics sometimes work, especially if you take a wide combination of bacteria in a high enough dose. But most of us will probably have to continue to take them for a very long time in order for the bacteria to maintain any permanent foothold in the gut. Studies on oral probiotics have so far been promising, but results are not consistent.

The list of clinical trials using probiotics is much longer than those using fecal transplants and includes: gastrointestinal function, irritable bowel syndrome, anxiety, depression, asthma, type 2 diabetes mellitus, hypertension, hyperlipidemia, alcoholic liver disease, rheumatoid arthritis, bacterial vaginosis, diverticular disease, respiratory infections in children, atopic dermatitis, fatty liver, lactose intolerance, coronary artery disease, bipolar disorder, antibiotic-associated diarrhea, hypertriglyceridemia, HIV, cancer, and necrotizing enterocolitis in preterm infants with very low body weight.

Our gut has its own ecology. And we know what can happen when people with great good intentions try to improve an environmental ecology. They add a new animal or plant in an attempt to resolve a specific problem, which then goes on to create many new problems. An ecology is far more complicated and harder to fix than we can imagine. The same is true with our gut.

Relationships among bacteria are intricate and not easy to figure out. It's too early to know which types of probiotic bacteria work for each particular disease. There are many factors yet to be understood, and most of the research has been done on animals. Human beings are inevitably far more complex, and results can be very different.

REFERENCES:

For information on clinical trials go to: https://clinicaltrials.gov/ and enter "fecal microbiome transplant" and "probiotics" in the search box.

Ridaura, VK et al., Gut microbiota from twins discordant for obesity modulate metabolism in mice. *Science* 2013 Sep 6; 341(6150):1241214.

Alang, N and Kelly, CR, Weight Gain After Fecal Microbiota Transplantation. *Open Forum Infect Dis* 2015; 2 (1): ofv004.

Konig, J et al., Consensus report: faecal microbiota transfer clinical applications and procedures. *Aliment Pharmacol Ther* 2017; 45: 222–239

Chu, ND et al., Profiling Living Bacteria Informs Preparation of Fecal Microbiota Transplantations. Zoetendal EG, ed. *PLoS ONE* 2017;12(1):e0170922.

Vermeire, S et al., Donor species richness determines faecal microbiota transplantation success in inflammatory bowel disease. *J Crohns Colitis* 2016; 10: 387–94. 54.

Van Nood, E et al., Duodenal infusion of donor feces for recurrent Clostridium difficile. *N Engl J Med* 2013; 368(5): 407–15.

Why Do Animals—Including Your Dog—Eat Poop? by Liz Langley, *National Geographic*, May 9, 2015

CHAPTER 2

Gut Feelings

What if you were seeing a psychiatrist, but instead of lying on a couch, talking about your feelings, and being prescribed a drug like Valium or Prozac, you were given a probiotic to take twice a day? Although it hasn't happened yet, the research suggests that it could and will. Of all the areas of research on gut bacteria, this one surprises me the most. I would never have suspected that our state of mind could be affected by the state of our gut bacteria. Yet recent animal studies have clearly shown that gut bacteria can alter anxiety, depression, and our body's response to stress.

Psychobiotic is a new scientific term to describe a probiotic that is used for mental health. How can a probiotic affect our mind? To answer this question, scientists again turned to animals and developed several models for studying the effects of gut bacteria on their mental health.

In one experiment, two groups of mice were fed two different kinds of broth. In one, researchers put a probiotic containing the friendly bacteria *Lactobacillus rhamnosus*. The mice were then tested in both a maze and a stress test, in which they were forced to swim in a tank with no escape. This is not a pleasant swim but is often used to test drugs for depression. The probiotic group of mice behaved completely differently from the control group. They were more willing to explore different areas of the maze, and less likely to give up and start floating when subjected to a forced swim. The addition of a single bacteria had completely changed their response to stress. The mice produced lower levels of the stress hormone cortisol and demonstrated an increase in the activity of an important chemical in the brain (gamma butyric acid or GABA), which can inhibit an overexcited nervous system.

In another experiment, researchers separated infant rats from their mothers, and then tested them with either antidepressant drugs or probiotics. All the separated pups initially showed poor performance on the forced swim test, as well as abnormal chemical changes in the brain. However, when some of the pups were given the probiotic *Bifidobacterium infantis*, they greatly improved. In fact, the mice that were given the probiotic did as well in the test as those given the antidepressant, suggesting that the probiotic acted as a true psychobiotic.

Human research involving psychobiotics is still at an early stage. Several studies have given subjects either probiotics or a placebo, and then tested them using self-reported effects on mood. Results have shown a significant improvement in positive moods and a decline in negativity. A reduction in cortisol was also found.

In one brain imaging study, subjects were first given either a psychobiotic mixture or a placebo. They were then shown images of frightened faces. The subjects taking the placebo showed a stress response in which some areas of the brain responsible for emotions became activated. Subjects receiving the psychobiotics showed less activity in these same areas of the brain, which suggests less vulnerability to stress.

These and other studies indicate that changing our gut bacteria really can affect emotional behavior, as well as memory. We will later see how gut bacteria affects social behavior and may play a critical role in certain neurological disorders such as autism and Alzheimer's disease.

Gut Rap Q & A:

H Bomb: What happens if all the psychos suddenly switch to yogurt instead of taking their meds?

Doc Gut: It's not a good idea for mental health patients to switch to yogurt. The research on animals, however, is very exciting. What it tells us is that the gut bacteria can communicate directly with the brain through neuronal and chemical pathways. But carefully controlled studies on humans are needed to determine the effectiveness of these programs.

Ms. Natural: Do all strains of probiotics work equally well?

Doc Gut: As I said, most of the findings are on animals, but it's clear that some bacteria strains do work better than others. And some work only for certain conditions.

H Bomb: What I want to know is: who's making all the money on these bug formulas?

Doc Gut: Good question. Many of the probiotics that are being studied have patents on them.

Ms. Natural: How can you patent Mother Nature?

Doc Gut: Different companies have created distinct strains of the bacteria, and have given them a specific name and number. This allows them to patent those bacteria.

H Bomb: But if the big drug companies are involved, there must be horrible side effects.

Doc Gut: Most of the studies have shown only positive effects on emotions and mental tasks. And although one preliminary human study showed a slight decline in memory, these results were not replicated.

Ms. Natural: How long does it take to get results with psychobiotics?

Doc Gut: No one is sure yet. The animal studies show that the effects of the psychobiotic on brain chemicals take about 2 to 4 weeks.

Ms. Natural: I'm wondering how this relates to the ancient wisdom of traditional health systems, which teaches us that diet can improve our mental and emotional state.

Doc Gut: The latest research findings fit very well with these time-tested concepts. Diet changes the composition of our gut bacteria. And we now know that changing the state of our gut bacteria can change our brain and many aspects of our mental health. What has not been scientifically studied yet is which diet is best for each condition.

REFERENCES:

Sarkar, A et al., Psychobiotics and the Manipulation of Bacteria–Gut–Brain Signals. *Trends in Neurosciences* November 2016; 39, (11), 763–781

Evrensel, A, and Ceylan, ME, The Gut-Brain Axis: The Missing Link in Depression. *Clinical Psychopharmacology and Neuroscience* 2015; 13(3): 239-244

Magnusson, KR et al., Relationships between diet-related changes in the gut microbiome and cognitive flexibility. *Neuroscience* 2015; 300:128-40

CHAPTER 3

Right From the Beginning

Have you ever wondered where your gut bacteria originated? Were they in you before you were born? Evidence indicates that we may be exposed to our mother's bacteria in the womb, but this is a debated topic.

We do know that it makes a big difference if a baby is born by caesarean birth, which is not uncommon. In a normal birth, the infant makes its journey down the birth canal and comes into contact with the mother's bacteria, which immediately begin to colonize the child's gut.

In a caesarean birth, the first exposure to bacteria is the mother's skin and the hospital environment, including the air of the operating room and the personal bacteria cloud of each of the attending doctors, nurses, and other staff. The problem is that hospitals are not as sterile as they are supposed to be and host some of the most dangerous bacteria in the world.

Many studies now show that children from caesarean births have a higher incidence of asthma, allergies, autoimmune diseases, and obesity. So it does matter whether we receive our mother's friendly bacteria or potentially lethal hospital bacteria.

It was my impression that caesarean births are relatively infrequent, but I was wrong. In some countries, like China, over 50% of all births are caesarean. And that's a lot of babies. In private hospitals in Brazil, the number reaches 80%. Italy has the second highest caesarean birth rate in Europe with 38%. In the US, over 30% of all births are caesarean.

The mother's birth canal is loaded with *Lactobacillus* bacteria, which is similar to the bacteria in yogurt. This and other early bacteria help to educate the immune system of the infant's gut about "good" and "bad" bacteria. If our immune system is deprived of this early education, we are far more likely to develop a wide range of diseases.

Gut Rap Q & A:

Ms. Natural: Why are there so many caesarean births?

Doc Gut: There are some important medical reasons including breech birth, twins, a previous caesarean section, or medical complications during pregnancy or labor. In Europe, doctors perceive the procedure as being safer since they can control the delivery date of the birth.

H Bomb: Hogwash! Doctors think a lot of themselves and they're not interested in being awakened in the middle of the night or being interrupted on the golf course to deliver a baby. Plus, by controlling the timing of the birth, they can slot them in, one after the other. Deliver more and make more money!

Ms. Natural: I heard about a new procedure for infants who are born by caesarean. It's called "gauze-in-the-vagina" technique.

Doc Gut: Yes. In this procedure, a piece of moist gauze is inserted into the mother's vagina about an hour before surgery. As soon as the child is born, the gauze is wiped all over their body, including the inside of the mouth, around the eyes, and the skin from head to toe.

H Bomb: Disgusting.

Doc Gut: Preliminary studies on C-section infants who have undergone this procedure show very good results. And the main types of bacteria in these babies are similar to those in infants who had a normal birth.

Ms. Natural: Is this procedure available everywhere?

Doc Gut: Doctors and medical institutions tend to be cautious, so it will take more research for it to be generally approved.

H Bomb: You're saying that it will take another 10 or 15 years of clinical trials before anyone benefits?

Doc Gut: Unfortunately, yes.

REFERENCES:

Arrieta, MC et al., The intestinal microbiome in early life: health and disease, *Frontiers in Immunology* September 2014; 5, 427

Mueller, NT et al., Prenatal exposure to antibiotics, cesarean section and risk of childhood obesity. *J Obes (Lond)* 2015; 39 (4): 665-670

Mesquita, DN et al., Cesarean Section Is Associated with Increased Peripheral and Central Adiposity in Young Adulthood: Cohort Study. *PLoS ONE* 2013; 8(6): e66827

Feehley, T et al., Microbial regulation of allergic responses to food. *Semin Immunopathol* September 2012; 34(5)

Wegienka, G et al., The Role of the Early-Life Environment in the Development of Allergic Disease. *Immunol Allergy Clin North Am* 2015; 35(1):1-17

CHAPTER 4

Antibiotics

Who hasn't taken antibiotics? I've taken them too many times! As a baby, they may well have saved my life. And as an adult traveling around the world, I survived some horribly unpleasant bouts of diarrhea by using antibiotics. When our kids had a bad earache or a flu, we took them to the doctor and they were prescribed antibiotics. They were everywhere.

There's no doubt that the widespread use of antibiotics starting in the 1950s was a major step in modern medicine and it has since saved millions of lives. In the past, childhood infections often resulted in early death, and for this alone, we are grateful for antibiotics. There is little doubt that they have dramatically increased people's lifespan, but most medical experts now agree that we have massively overprescribed these wonder drugs, and there is a worldwide movement to limit their usage.

Bacteria are adaptable little critters and one of the most pressing problems of the overuse of antibiotics is the development of antibiotic-resistant bacteria. According to the Centers for Disease Control and Prevention, at least 2 million people in the

US become infected every year with bacteria that are resistant to antibiotics, and at least 23,000 people die as a direct result of untreatable infections.

In the past, no one had a clue that antibiotics would lead to the massive disruption of friendly gut bacteria. Now that we realize how important our gut bacteria are, scientists have become extremely wary of the long-term effects of antibiotics. A single dose of one antibiotic is like an atomic bomb, wiping out trillions of mostly friendly bacteria. And when we finish a course of antibiotic treatment, the composition of our gut bacteria is vastly different from before. Normally, we have over 1000 different types of bacteria living in our gut, but antibiotics wipe out entire populations, causing us to lose bacterial diversity that is important for our health!

Even if, by some miracle, you've never taken an antibiotic, it is almost certain that you will be exposed to them if you eat meat. For over 50 years, farmers have been giving low doses of antibiotics to animals to increase their weight. (More weight means more money.) Unless you are a strict vegetarian, you are probably ingesting some antibiotics every time you eat meat, unless you specifically purchase antibiotic-free meat. Studies have shown that antibiotics are also present in the groundwater of rural areas.

We know that disrupting the gut bacteria is not a good thing. But there may be times when antibiotics are the only viable choice. Most doctors today will recommend that you take probiotics to reseed your gut after a course of antibiotics, even though it is not certain if this is enough to restore your optimal gut health.

Gut Rap Q & A:

Ms. Natural: I heard an antibiotic destroys all bacteria in our gut. Is this true?

Doc Gut: They don't kill all the bacteria, but they wipe out a substantial percentage, especially friendly bacteria, and it may take several years before they are fully restored.

Ms. Natural: Can we replenish our bacteria by eating yogurt or other probiotics?

Doc Gut: No. There are over 1000 different types of bacteria in our gut, and no probiotic has remotely that many bacteria in it. We don't yet know how to replace all the good gut bacteria that are wiped out by antibiotics. It is possible that some are still present but in very small numbers.

Ms. Natural: Soil contains many bacteria and when they are killed by pesticides or other toxins all we need to do is to allow the soil to rest for a few years and the bacteria return.

Doc Gut: It's a good analogy, especially since soil bacteria play such an important role in the growth of plants. It may well be that after a few years our gut bacteria are able to completely grow back. It depends on how they were wiped out in the first place. Even soil has a hard time recovering when it has been napalmed. Some antibiotics behave like napalm in the gut, with devastating effect. And if they are taken over months or years, it's difficult to know how long a full recovery might take.

H Bomb: Bacteria are not smart, right? After all, we're talking about one of the simplest forms of life.

Doc Gut: This simple form of life has existed for some 3.5 billion years. Whether we call them smart or not, they can adapt to many different environments, from extreme heat to extreme cold. They can also pass information to other bacteria. For instance, if one type of bacteria finds a way to avoid an antibiotic, it is able to pass this information to another bacteria. This exchange of knowledge occurs by means of the transfer of genes, which allows them to constantly change and adapt. This is especially true in hospitals, where they have been attacked by strong antibiotics, and have had to become more adaptive.

The first appearance of penicillin-resistant bacteria occurred in the 1950s. In the 1960s, methicillin-resistant *Staphylococcus aureus* (MRSA) emerged. A new antibiotic, vancomycin, was introduced in the 1970s, and again bacteria became resistant to it. The newest "smart" bacteria are carbapenem-resistant *Enterobacteriaceae* or CRE, a very powerful bacteria that is resistant to even the latest antibiotics. The medical profession knows that it's losing the race and is searching for new solutions.

Ms. Natural: Before the discovery of antibiotics how did they fight infection?

Doc Gut: There were many different approaches and one of them was to use good bacteria to fight the bad ones. *Bacillus subtilis*, for example, was used in WWII to fight dysentery. In North Africa, hundreds of German soldiers began to die each week due to dysentery. The Germans noticed that the native Arabs protected themselves by eating horse or camel dung, so they organized a group of scientists to investigate the situation. The scientists reasoned that there must be a natural substance in the dung, and when it was examined closely, they found that it was full of *B. subtilis*. They then figured out how to culture the bacteria and gave it to their troops. The dysentery was stopped. This same bacteria is used in foods in Japan and in probiotics in the US.

Another example is a bacteria called *Bdellovibrio bacteriovorus*. Recent research in England suggests that this may be a new solution to an antibiotic-resistant strain of bacteria known as *Shigella flexneri*, a common cause of food poisoning. The *Shigella* bacteria contaminates food and causes havoc in the gut. Because it has become antibiotic-resistant, patients have to live with diarrhea and wait until their body can cure itself.

At present, only animal research has been done on the effects of *Bdellovibrio*. The findings suggest that it is a dominant predator of other bacteria and can kill *Shigella* by breaking it apart from the inside. When it does this, white blood cells are automatically stimulated to destroy the bacteria. Other predatory bacteria are being researched as a means of fighting the ever-increasing number of new antibiotic-resistant bacteria.

Ms. Natural: What is the effect of prenatal antibiotics?

Doc Gut: This is an area of great concern. In one large study, mothers who were given antibiotics during the second or third trimester had children with a much higher risk of obesity, compared to those who did not receive antibiotics.

REFERENCES:

Francino, MP, Antibiotics and the Human Gut Microbiome: Dysbioses and Accumulation of Resistances. *Frontiers in Microbiology* January 2016; 6, 1543

Mueller, NT et al., Prenatal exposure to antibiotics, cesarean section and risk of childhood obesity. *Int J Obes (Lond)* April 2015; 39(4): 665–670

Willis, AR et al., Injections of Predatory Bacteria Work Alongside Host Immune Cells to Treat Shigella Infection in Zebrafish Larvae. *Current Biology* December 2016; 26, 24, 3343–3351

Perez-Cobas, AE et al., Gut microbiota disturbance during antibiotic therapy: a multi-omic approach. *Gut* Nov 2013; 62(11),1591-601

Ventola, CL, The Antibiotic Resistance Crisis: Part 1: Causes and Threats. *Pharmacy and Therapeutics* 2015; 40(4):277-283.

One example of a report on antibiotics in groundwater in Minnesota is available at: http://pubs.usgs.gov/sir/2014/5096/pdf/sir2014-5096.pdf

CHAPTER 5

Diet and Lifestyle

Our gut bacteria are strongly influenced by our diet. This makes perfect sense since the foods we eat ultimately feed our gut bacteria. And our first food is milk, either from our mother's breast or from a bottle containing some formula. Scientists can immediately see the effects of these two diets by analyzing the different types of bacteria that come from them.

We know from research that human breast milk offers a number of advantages. The colostrum part of the breast milk, for example, contains immunoglobulins that can defend against various bad microorganisms. These include IgM, IgG, and IgA, which help to protect the child while his or her immune system is developing. IgA also contributes to the growth of our friendly gut bacteria.

One of the most unusual advantages of breast milk has to do with the complex sugars it contains called oligosaccharides. These compounds are also present in cow's milk, but human milk contains a larger quantity and wider variety.

Oligosaccharides can't be digested and absorbed in our small intestine so why does a mother go to the work of making them in her breast milk? The answer is interesting. These sugars are made for the nourishment of one type of bacteria, which lives in the large intestine. These bacteria are called *Bifidobacterium infantis,* and they are very helpful for the proper development of the baby's gut.

B. infantis makes sure that the cell lining of an infant's gut is tightly sealed. If the bacteria is not present, many health problems can occur. Studies show, for example, that formula-fed babies have significantly more inflammation and gut permeability than breastfed babies. Research further suggests that formula-fed babies have an increased risk of obesity in later childhood.

This is only the beginning of the story. Once the child switches from breast milk to solid foods, there is another change in the composition of the gut bacteria. This change stabilizes at about three years old, and can stay fairly constant for most of our lives. When we reach our elderly years, the types and numbers of bacteria decrease, which is not ideal for our health. However, if we at any time in our lives decide to make a big change in our diet, for example, switching from a meat diet to a vegetarian diet, the composition of gut bacteria will change in a matter of days. The reason for this is, again, that different types of gut bacteria prefer different types of food we eat. Some like meat, while others favor fiber.

Diet isn't the only thing that can change our gut bacteria. There are many other factors, including antibiotics, infection, and environmental and lifestyle changes. Research in Germany, for example, showed that mice that were exposed to cigarette smoke over a 24-week period had a significant shift in the composition of their gut bacteria. This is particularly interesting because cigarette smoke is a known risk factor in inflammatory bowel diseases like Crohn's Disease. A study done on humans also showed a change in gut bacteria composition after the cessation of smoking, with an overall increase in gut bacteria diversity, which would indicate a healthier gut.

Can exercise affect gut bacteria? It does. A study in Ireland compared professional athletes with others who exercised lightly or hardly at all. The professional athletes were all shown to have greater diversity of a family of bacteria known as *Akkermansiaceae*. Research has linked this type of bacteria to a decreased risk for obesity and inflammation throughout the body. Other studies have found that exercise helps by reducing the bad effects of a high-fat diet.

What about stress? Yes, stress has a bad effect on gut bacteria and the entire digestive system. We will talk more about it later.

Gut Rap Q & A:

Ms. Natural: Is dietary fiber as important as the health magazines say?

Doc Gut: Dietary fiber is a very important part of a healthy diet. Studies show that it is both preventive and therapeutic for bowel disorders and other conditions, such as heart disease or obesity. In the process of digesting fiber, the gut bacteria produce beneficial by-products, which include a group of compounds called short-chained fatty acids or SCFAs. Studies show that SCFAs have many benefits, including providing energy to the cells lining the lower bowels. They also enter the bloodstream and produce positive effects on other cells in the body.

Ms. Natural: How do different diets affect our gut bacteria?

Doc Gut: No one is sure yet. Several different studies have attempted to look at how carbohydrates, fats, and proteins affect the gut bacteria. High-fat diets, for example, induce an increase in certain substances from bacteria, such as lipopolysaccharides or LPS. These may increase intestinal permeability and cause inflammation. Other studies suggest that high-fat diets can change our bacterial composition and cause obesity. The degree to which long-term dietary patterns can create change in gut bacteria is still being researched and debated.

Ms. Natural: What about a gluten-free diet?

Doc Gut: One study examined the effects of a gluten-free diet over a one-month period. The most interesting change was a decrease in a family of bacteria called *Veillonellaceae*. This is a type of bacteria that tends to increase inflammation and is found to be higher in patients with bowel disorders.

H Bomb: I'll bet that the gut bacteria in the US are better than those in any other country in the world!

Doc Gut: Not really. People living in more primitive areas such as the jungles of Africa have a greater diversity of gut bacteria than those of us living in developed countries. Gut bacteria changes with geography. To a large extent, this may be due to the amounts of fiber in the diet of a particular region.

H Bomb: Big deal, so people in developing countries have more types of gut bacteria than we do. What does it mean anyway?

Doc Gut: It is a big deal. Greater diversity of bacteria tends to be a sign of good health. Gut bacteria produce many bioactive compounds, and we know that some of these have an important effect on health. The good gut bacteria can protect us from the bad ones. There's a war constantly going on in our gut. The good bacteria and the bad bacteria are competing for food. We want to do everything we possibly can to help the good guys win the war. There are many advantages, as we will learn, of having a healthy population of gut bacteria.

REFERENCES:

Conlon, MA, and Bird, AR, The Impact of Diet and Lifestyle on Gut Microbiota and Human Health. *Nutrients* 2015; 7, 17-44

O'Sullivan, A et al., The Influence of Early Infant-Feeding Practices on the Intestinal Microbiome and Body Composition in Infants. *Nutrition and Metabolic Insights* 2015;8(S1) 1–9

Clarke, SF et al., Exercise and associated dietary extremes impact on gut microbial diversity. *Gut* Dec 2014; 63(12):1913-20

Biedermann, L et al., Smoking Cessation Induces Profound Changes in the Composition of the Intestinal Microbiota in Humans. *PLoS ONE* 2013; 8(3): e59260.

Bonder, MJ et al., The influence of a short-term gluten-free diet on the human gut microbiome. *Genome Medicine* 2016; 8:45

Allais, L et al., Chronic cigarette smoke exposure induces microbial and inflammatory shifts and mucin changes in the murine gut. *Environ Microbiol* May 2016; 18(5):1352-63

Cani, PD et al., Endotoxemia-Induced Inflammation in High-Fat Diet–Induced Obesity and Diabetes in Mice. *Diabetes* 2008; 57:1470–1481,

Campbell, SC et al., The Effect of Diet and Exercise on Intestinal Integrity and Microbial Diversity in Mice. *PLoS ONE* Mar 2016; 11(3):e0150502.

Evans, CC et al., Exercise prevents weight gain and alters the gut microbiota in a mouse model of high fat diet-induced obesity. *PLoS ONE* Mar 2014; 9(3):e92193.

Le Chatelier, E et al., Richness of human gut microbiome correlates with metabolic markers. *Nature* 2013; 500(7464):541-6

Monda, V et al., Exercise Modifies the Gut Microbiota with Positive Health Effects. *Oxid Med Cell Longev* 2017; 2017:3831972

CHAPTER 6

The Cloud Around You

In 2007, researchers from the human microbiome project estimated that there are about 100 trillion microorganisms in and on the body. Newer research has revised this number to about 30 trillion.

The numbers not only change, but can also be confusing. For example, the human microbiome project reported there are over 10,000 different types of microorganisms, but the vast majority of these are about 1000 different types of bacteria living in our lower gut. Our stomach, with its acidic climate, is not a popular neighborhood; neither is the small intestine, teeming with digestive enzymes.

Some numbers can be alarming. For example, in one intimate 10-second kiss, over 80 million bacteria are exchanged! Gut bacteria have 8 million genes, 360 times more genes than the human body does. There are more microorganisms living on our hands than people living on the planet.

Every time we touch anything, or anyone, our skin comes into contact with a vast number of microorganisms. These microorganisms thrive almost everywhere on the surface of the skin but they favor proximity to a sweat gland. For bacteria, this is like living next to a convenience store, where water and fatty acids snacks are readily available. Good bacteria on our skin act as our private security forces, creating antimicrobial substances that protect us from the bad guys.

In addition to bacteria, other microorganisms live on and in us, such as fungi, viruses, and yeast. Fungi can take up residence on our feet and cause athlete's foot. For men, they can also locate themselves around the genital area and cause a long-term fungal infection. For women, a form of fungi can overpopulate the vagina, causing a *Candida* yeast infection.

In most cases, the different microorganisms such as bacteria, viruses, fungi, and yeast compete for supremacy. In the vagina, for example, *L. acidophilus*, a friendly type of bacteria, will fight off yeast and help create a healthy environment.

We can try to control our exposure to microbes by staying at home and regularly washing our hands and wiping everything down with antimicrobial products. But if you ever take any public form of transportation, a bus, plane, or train, there is no avoiding microorganisms (The Good, the Bad, and the Ugly). Studies mapping out the varieties of microorganisms in a subway found vast numbers of many different types, some of which haven't even been classified yet.

Picture yourself walking down a city street. It is as if you, and everyone else, are surrounded by a cloud of microbes, and each time you come in contact with another person ("Thank you, Ma'am." "Excuse me, Sir.") you exchange microbes.

No matter how germaphobic we may be, short of living in a hazmat suit or a bubble, we can't avoid them. From the very beginning, as the infant passes through the birth canal, he or she receives important friendly ones. Mother passes on more from her skin, her kisses and caresses. And when she takes the baby outside for fun in the sun the child is exposed to new microbes. Everyone knows it is almost impossible to stop children from touching or putting things into their mouth. When we look away for a moment, they will eat dirt, filled with a whole new array of microorganisms. Some doctors and scientists, in fact, advocate bringing up children in rural environments where they can be exposed to new bacteria.

The "hygiene hypothesis" argues that our super hygienic environment is hurting us. Our immune system is not exposed to enough different microorganisms and does not have an opportunity to adapt and become fully educated. As a result, we are more prone to allergies, asthma, and infections.

For the first time it is possible to measure the different types of bacteria in our gut and other areas of our body. It's even affordable. A stool, skin, or mouth sample can be mailed to a commercial laboratory that will analyze it and send you back a report. I chose to use the American Gut Project because it is part of a large scientific experiment. The instructions are fairly straightforward and once you receive the results, you can compare yourself with others in the study. I had ten times more *Prevotella* bacteria than others. Is this good or bad? It's probably good, and normal for me since I am a vegetarian and these bacteria like veggies and fiber. I didn't do the samples for either skin or mouth. (I was, however, tempted to do the gut test for our dog.)

Gut Rap Q & A:

H Bomb: I hate microbes. When I travel, I never drink the water; I don't eat any food that isn't well cooked or can't be peeled, and I use antimicrobial wipes at all times.

Doc Gut: It's important to take precautions when we are traveling, especially in developing countries where sanitation isn't always good. Our immune systems have not been exposed to the microorganisms in these places, so it's easy for us to come down with Delhi belly or Montezuma's revenge.

The problem is that unfriendly microorganisms are transferred by hand (literally) to the food we eat. If the food isn't well cooked, we can become overwhelmed by microbes to which we have little or no immunity, and some are more dangerous than others.

H Bomb: Finally we agree on something! What about the subway research? I always hated subways, but the findings you're talking about make them hot zones!

Doc Gut: Microorganisms are everywhere and it's impossible to completely avoid them. In a subway, however, we receive an extra big dose since so many people are exposed to each other's microbes in a confined space.

H Bomb: But the bad guys can be destroyed, right? Take the smallpox virus—it used to be everywhere, and now it's been eliminated.

Doc Gut: Smallpox is thought to have been around for about 50,000 years, since before the beginning of civilization. At the end of the

18th century, it killed 400,000 Europeans annually. In the 20th century, between 300 and 500 million people died from this disease. In 1979 the World Health Organization (WHO) proclaimed the global eradication of smallpox, through the worldwide use of the smallpox vaccination. As far as we know, the only place smallpox still exists is in carefully guarded laboratories.

Ms. Natural: Is everyone's gut bacteria different?

Doc Gut: Yes. The latest research suggests that each of us has a unique combination of bacteria in our gut as well as on our skin, in our mouth, and other areas. And as we mentioned, the combination of microbes can change due to factors like age, diet, environment, and lifestyle.

Ms. Natural: What can I do to make sure that the combination of bacteria in my body is healthy?

Doc Gut: Diet and lifestyle are probably the two most important factors. If we wipe out one particular type by taking an antibiotic, we can take a probiotic, but it's unclear how well that works. Analyzing the parts of an ecological system does not give us an understanding of the whole. A great deal more research needs to be done, and ancient health practices need to be reexamined, especially to determine the right diet for each individual.

REFERENCES:

Turnbaugh, PJ et al., The human microbiome project: exploring the microbial part of ourselves in a changing world. *Nature.* 2007; 449(7164):804-810

The University of Maryland Medical Center has an amazing database. This page gives a comprehensive summary of the beneficial effects of *L. acidophilus*: http://umm.edu/health/medical/altmed/supplement lactobacillus-acidophilus.

Information on the American Gut Project can be found at http://www.americangut.org.

See Wikipedia for more on smallpox.

CHAPTER 7

The Business of Gut Bacteria

When I mentioned some new gut research to a friend, his comment was, "Sure, I hear it's the next cure for cancer." This response didn't surprise me. I get it. All kinds of popular articles say that altering our gut bacteria cures virtually everything. Let's step back for a moment and forget the sensational articles. Instead, let's look at some clearly established things that gut bacteria do.

First, gut bacteria help us digest food. This includes the fibrous foods doctors are always recommending. The bacteria in the lower gut have the necessary enzymes in them to break down these fibers and make them ready for fermentation. Some of the important products of this fermentation are short-chain fatty acids (SCFAs) like acetic acid, propionic acid, and butyric acid—a primary source of nutrients and energy for cells lining the colon. SCFAs have many other functions, including helping the body absorb essential minerals like calcium, magnesium, and iron.

Second, our gut bacteria makes B vitamins, including thiamine or B_1, riboflavin or B_2, nicotinic acid (a form of niacin) or B_3, pantothenic acid or B_5, pyridoxine or B_6, biotin or B_7, folate (folic acid) or B_9, and cobalamin or B_{12}, as well as a certain type of vitamin K, which is necessary to make special blood clotting factors.

We are not yet certain who benefits the most from these vitamins, our gut or our entire body. Vitamin B_{12} is an interesting example. It's involved in the metabolism of every cell in our body, and it is especially important to the functioning of our nervous system and the formation of red blood cells. The human body cannot produce vitamin B_{12}, and neither can any animal, fungi, or plant. This vitamin can only be made by bacteria and by archaea (microorganisms that are a little more advanced than bacteria). Vitamin B_{12} deficiency is often seen in people who don't eat meat, fish, or dairy products. As a result, scientists have suggested that the gut bacteria alone are not capable of fulfilling our B_{12} needs and that dietary vitamins are required. The production of B_{12} in the gut, therefore, is probably more important for the health of the cells in the colon rather than for the rest of our body.

A third important function of the gut bacteria is to help protect our body from the invasion of harmful microorganisms. Approximately 70-80% of our total immune system is located in the lining of the gut and the friendly gut bacteria help the immune system in a number of different ways. Certain bacteria can, for example, produce chemicals that fend off bad bacteria, and the friendly bacteria also occupy critical locations along the gut lining so that bad bacteria do not have access.

The gut immune system is called GALT, which stands for gut-associated lymphoid tissue. Some of the immune cells have the ability to sample microbes inside the gut to determine if they are good or bad. If a bad guy is detected, other immune cells in the lining will be alerted to react. GALT is a kind of early warning defense system, which produces a wide range of antimicrobial chemicals that destroy harmful pathogens and stimulate other immune cells to prepare for imminent attack. Our friendly gut bacteria work with the GALT defense system to help protect the gut lining.

Fourth, gut bacteria are critical to the full development of the gut lining and its many different cells. Experiments on germ-free mice (strange animals in all respects) show that without gut bacteria critical immune cells in the GALT system do not develop properly. Also, nerve cells in the gut lining develop abnormally, with reduced levels of certain key neurotransmitters that may be important for the development of the entire gut nervous system.

Fifth, gut bacteria communicate with our brain and influence, among other things, our digestion, appetite, and state of mind. They are part of the gut-brain axis, which we will talk about later.

Sixth, an abnormal composition of gut bacteria seem to be involved in many different types of diseases, such as: inflammatory bowel disease, irritable bowel syndrome, colon cancer, allergies, asthma, autoimmune diseases, Parkinson's disease, autism, Alzheimer's, multiple sclerosis, depression, anxiety, types 1 and 2 diabetes, stroke, high blood pressure, high cholesterol, and heart disease. The list grows longer every day.

My friend was right. Gut bacteria are often misrepresented as a magic bullet for serious diseases like cancer, but this in no way diminishes their importance. We have to wait (impatiently) until definitive clinical trials are completed, but in the meantime, we can enjoy this exciting field as it reveals one of nature's remarkable hidden mysteries.

Gut Rap Q & A:

Ms. Natural: What other functions do the bacteria have?

Doc Gut: We are just now learning about the many thousands of chemicals they produce and how the measurement and use of these compounds might be useful for the diagnosis and treatment of different disorders.

Ms. Natural: Can you give some examples?

Doc Gut: In addition to vitamins and short-chained fatty acids, there are organic acids, amino acids, secondary bile acids, components of lipid transport, and important chemical messengers. There is an entire field of gut bacteria metabolomics that focuses on the measurement and analysis of these substances.

H Bomb: But not everything bacteria produce is good. What about the bad stuff?

Doc Gut: Certain harmful bacteria, as we will soon learn, produce super toxins. Accidentally ingesting them results in food poisoning, which can be lethal in some cases.

H Bomb: What about smelly gas?

Doc Gut: Bacteria produce different types of gas, such as methane, hydrogen, and carbon dioxide. It's a normal part of the process of fermentation in the lower gut. We all know that too much gas causes discomfort, bloating, or pain, which we will talk more about when we discuss irritable bowel syndrome (IBS).

REFERENCES:

For a complete list of functions see Gut Flora at Wikipedia.

Conlon, MA and Bird, AR, The Impact of Diet and Lifestyle on Gut Microbiota and Human Health. *Nutrients* 2015; 7, 17-44

Yano, JM et al., Indigenous Bacteria from the Gut Microbiota Regulate Host Serotonin Biosynthesis. *Cell* 2015; 161 (2) 264-276

Degnan, PH et al., Vitamin B12 as a modulator of gut microbial ecology. *Cell Metabolism* 2014; 20(5):769-778

Rossi, M et al., Folate Production by Probiotic Bacteria. *Nutrients* 2011; 3(1):118-134

Vernocchi, P et al., Gut Microbiota Profiling: Metabolomics Based Approach to Unravel Compounds Affecting Human Health. *Front Microbiol* Jul 2016; 7:1144

CHAPTER 8

The Good, the Bad, and the Vile:
PART 1

First, the Good Guys

Let's take a quick look at some of the friendly or good bacteria that occupy our gut. These are the heroes in our body's ongoing battle against sickness. We've already mentioned one of our most well-known warriors, *Lactobacillus acidophilus*. Its name comes from the Latin roots *lacto*, which means milk, and *acido philus*, which mean acid-loving. The genus *Lactobacillus* is among the most useful bacteria in the lower gut and vagina.

L. acidophilus produces both hydrogen peroxide and lactic acid, which inhibit the growth of harmful bacteria and other harmful microorganisms. Clinical trials show that this bacteria can help treat ulcerative colitis, vaginal infection, and a wide variety of other health conditions.

Another friendly bacteria is the species *Lactobacillus plantarum*, found in fermented foods such as sauerkraut, dill pickles, and kimchi. It has been used to treat gut disorders, and can reduce the growth of gas-producing bacteria in our intestines. One very interesting study discovered that after the introduction of *L. plantarum,* there was an increase in an important nerve growth factor located in a critical area of the brain involved in memory and emotions. The researchers suggest that this bacteria may have a positive effect in the treatment of depression. It has also been thought to have a therapeutic role in the treatment of HIV.

Lactobacillus rhamnosus occurs naturally in the gut and is often found in probiotics. When it was isolated from the gut of a healthy patient in 1983, it was patented by two doctors with the initials GG. As a result, the strain is sometimes called *L. rhamnosus* GG or LGG. With over 800 studies, LGG is at this moment the most widely studied probiotic bacteria in the world. Findings include its ability to stick to the mucous membrane of the intestines, restore the balance of gut bacteria, diminish the production of toxic compounds by other intestinal bacteria, and enhance the immune response during infection. Other benefits of LGG include helping to relieve allergic reactions to peanuts in children, the prevention and treatment of various types of diarrhea, lowering the risk of respiratory tract infection in children attending day-care, and reducing anxiety.

Bifidobacterium infantis is one of 32 species that are part of the *Bifidobacterium* genus, commonly used in probiotics. It is one of the first bacteria to populate an infant's gut, and, as we discussed earlier, breast milk contains a complex sugar that specifically nourishes this bacteria. Its beneficial effects include the ability to protect against bad bacteria, help digest certain food products, promote anti-inflammatory activity, and produce certain vitamins. Randomized controlled trials of probiotics in premature infants have shown that *B. infantis* decreases the risk of necrotizing enterocolitis more than other probiotics. Necrotizing enterocolitis is a life-threatening disease in premature infants, which is caused by damage to the intestinal tissue. *B. infantis* is also effective in relieving symptoms of irritable bowel syndrome (IBS).

Finally, we have the friendly bacteria *Streptococcus thermophiles*. The word *Streptococcus* comes from a Greek term that means easily bent and refers to the way the bacterium is grouped in chains resembling a twisted string of beads. *Thermophilus* means love of heat and refers to the bacteria's ability to thrive at high temperatures. Studies have been conducted to test the health benefits of *S. thermophiles,* and it has been found to reduce symptoms of ulcerative colitis.

Gut Rap Q & A:

**H Bomb: Are there other good guys besides
the ones you mentioned?**

Doc Gut: There are many more. In fact, good guys outnumber bad guys 10 to 1. Most of the bacteria discovered in the gut are good guys.

**Ms. Natural: With these odds, why do so many people
suffer from painful stomach and gut problems?**

Doc Gut: Some of the bad guys are really bad. And when we use antibiotics to counter pathogens, many friendly gut bacteria can be disrupted or destroyed, causing long-term problems in our gut health.

**Ms. Natural: Can you give other examples of probiotic bacteria,
especially the ones that produce good effects?**

Doc Gut: *Lactobacillus reuteri* is a bacteria that inhabits the gut of both humans and animals. It is commonly found in probiotic formulas. A commercial company has patented several well-researched strains. Among the many findings are that *L. reuteri* produces certain substances that have beneficial effects on our physiology. One of these substances, reuterin, inhibits the growth of harmful Gram-negative and Gram-positive bacteria, and is as effective as the antibiotic gentamicin in preventing *E. coli*-related deaths. It can prevent the growth of yeasts, fungi, and protozoa, and can reduce *Helicobacter pylori*, which can cause peptic ulcers.

It is also used in the prevention and treatment of diarrhea in children, the treatment of infant colic, and to alleviate necrotizing enterocolitis in preterm infants.

Ms. Natural: Which probiotic do you recommend?

Doc Gut: That's a question I'm still researching. There are so many new probiotics on the market each day, and both the dosage and number of types of bacteria keep improving. Go to docgut.com to see the latest evaluations.

REFERENCES:

Ghouri, YA et al., Systematic review of randomized controlled trials of probiotics, prebiotics, and synbiotics in inflammatory bowel disease. *Clin Exp Gastroenterol* December 2014; 7: 473–487

Saez-Lara, MJ et al., The Role of Probiotic Lactic Acid Bacteria and Bifidobacteria in the Prevention and Treatment of Inflammatory Bowel Disease and Other Related Diseases: A Systematic Review of Randomized Human Clinical Trials. *Biomed Res Int (Systematic review)* 2015; 15

Andrieu, JM et al., Mucosal SIV vaccines comprising inactivated virus particles and bacterial adjuvants induce CD8+ T-regulatory cells that suppress SIV-positive CD4+ T-cell activation and prevent SIV infection in the macaque model. *Front. Immunol* 2014; 5: 297

For more details on the scientific finding for different bacteria, please see docgut.com.

CHAPTER 9

The Good, the Bad, and the Vile:
PART 2

Now For The Bad Guys

Clostridium botulinum is certainly one of the bad guys, and produces a number of super toxins. Ingesting even the tiniest amount (equivalent to five grains of sand) of this toxin blocks nerve function and causes muscle paralysis, which can lead to death. *C. botulinum* also has nasty relatives like *C. difficile*, which causes severe and often fatal diarrhea. Yet not all of the over 100 different types of *Clostridium* are bad. Some are friendly and help cure digestive disorders. To make it even more interesting, *C. botulinum* produces the toxin that is commercially used in Botox!

Salmonella is another bad bacteria that frequently causes food poisoning. Children are the most susceptible to *Salmonella*, but anyone can become sick. In the battle between good and bad bacteria, numbers count. Our stomach acid kills some bad bacteria, but many make their way to the gut where they wreak havoc on our digestive lining. Every year, over a million people in the US are affected by food poisoning from *Salmonella*. A less common variety of *Salmonella* causes typhoid fever.

Shigella is a bad bacteria that is closely related to *Salmonella*. It's one of the leading causes of diarrhea worldwide, resulting in 160 million cases of diarrhea and over half a million deaths every year.

Listeria monocytogenes is responsible for 1,600 illnesses and 260 deaths in the US annually, but it can cause meningitis in newborns. This is why pregnant mothers are advised to avoid certain soft cheeses that are often contaminated. It's interesting that both the bacteria and the mouthwash are named after Sir John Lister (1827-1912).

The list goes on. *Staphylococcus aureus* is a common cause of respiratory and skin infection, as well as food poisoning. This is another bacteria that can either be harmful or friendly. The harmful strains produce powerful toxins that disrupt gut function. We have already mentioned the newest and most serious problem, the evolution of antibiotic-resistant strains of *Staphylococcus aureus* or methicillin-resistant *S. aureus* (MRSA), which are unfortunately most often encountered in hospitals.

Escherichia coli (*E. coli*) is a rod-shaped bacteria that is normally friendly and helps with the function of the digestive system. Some strains, however, can disrupt the lining of the gut and cause severe diarrhea. If *E. coli* gets into the blood, it can lead to severe illness and even death.

What about the truly vile bacteria? It's hard to pick a #1.

We could start with the ones that have killed the most people. In Europe during the 14th century, *Yersinia pestis* caused Bubonic plague or Black Death, which resulted in the death of half of all the people living there (about 25 million). This bacteria is carried by fleas, which at some point leave their rodent host and bite a human. The bacteria then enters the bloodstream, causing a full-blown infection, which more than half the time results in death.

And Bubonic plague is still around. Even in the US, a few people become infected every year. During October 2016, five people were infected in Colorado, four in New Mexico, two in California, two in Arizona, one in Oregon, and one in Utah. Larger outbreaks occur in other parts of the world, but now that it is possible to treat the infection, it does not spread as in the past.

If we were to pick the bacteria that carries the greatest stigma, it would have to be *Mycobacterium leprae,* the bacteria that causes leprosy. It destroys nerves and the patient loses his or her sense of touch, with parts of the body becoming numb and easily injured. Diminishing eyesight, secondary infection, and deformity can also occur. Historically, this disfiguring disease was accompanied by a horror of contamination, and patients were banished from their homes and communities and exiled to isolated colonies. In the modern age, an effective treatment is offered for free by the World Health Organization (WHO).

Vibrio cholera, the bacteria responsible for cholera, is even today, high in the category of vile bacteria. Highly contagious, it affects 3 to 5 million people in developing countries, particularly children, and causes about 100,000 deaths each year. It is spread mostly by means of contaminated water.

Our last vile candidate is *Bacillus anthracis,* which causes anthrax. In the past, this disease killed hundreds of thousands of people and animals. Today, only 2,000 cases worldwide are reported annually, and about 2 in the US. The main reason we classify this bacteria as vile is its potential for use in biological warfare.

Gut Rap Q & A

H Bomb: Are viruses worse than bacteria?

Doc Gut: Viruses can be very ugly. I mentioned the smallpox virus, which killed hundred of millions of people in the past, including an appallingly high percentage of native people in North and South America. And HIV continues to cause suffering throughout the world even though effective treatments are available in some countries.

H Bomb: What's the most deadly virus?

Doc Gut: Most experts agree that the *Marburg* and the *Ebola* viruses are the most virulent. These viruses cause severe bleeding of mucous membranes, skin, and organs, killing 90% of those infected. There are other deadly viruses that we may not have heard about such as the *Machupo* virus, *Kyasanur Forest* virus, *Junin* virus, *Crimea-Congo* fever virus, *Hantavirus*, and *Lassa* virus.

Ms. Natural: What about the *Zika* virus?

Doc Gut: The *Zika* virus has recently received a great deal of publicity. In adults, it generally causes only mild symptoms, similar to a minor form of dengue fever. Like many other diseases, it is transmitted by mosquitoes. The most serious problem with the *Zika* virus is that it can also spread from a pregnant woman to her fetus, resulting in serious brain malformation.

H Bomb: I read somewhere that bacteria might just be puppets that are controlled by viruses.

Doc Gut: There are some viruses that actually live inside the bacteria cells. One of these is called *crAssphage*, and it's present in about three-quarters of gut bacteria in people all over the world. Is it the "puppet master" of the gut bacteria? Nobody knows, but there is an intensive investigation into *crAssphage* and other viruses. The human virome is a term that describes all the viruses that are both in and on us, and includes the genes within the viruses.

Ms. Natural: What about chickenpox or measles?

Doc Gut: Chickenpox is caused by a virus known as *Varicella zoster virus* (VZV). It is an airborne disease, which is highly contagious. Every year, many millions are infected with either chickenpox or shingles (*herpes zoster*). Shingles is caused by a reactivation of the chickenpox virus, which is somehow able to remain dormant in the nerve cells for a long time, even years. No one is clear about how it does this.

Measles is also caused by an airborne virus and is highly contagious. Although it usually resolves itself, there can be severe complications. This disease affects about 20 million people a year. In 2013 the number of deaths worldwide was less than 100,000, which is a huge improvement considering that in 1980 it was estimated to have killed several million. Children are the most susceptible, and those who are malnourished are especially at risk for death.

Ms. Natural: What about Lyme disease?

Doc Gut: Lyme disease is caused by a spirochete bacteria of the genus *Borrelia*. Transmitted to humans by the bite of infected ticks, it can hide in the cells of the infected person for many years, eventually causing severe problems in the joints, heart, or brain, as well as other parts of the body. It is especially debilitating if not treated at an early stage.

H Bomb: Tell us about flesh-eating bacteria!

Doc Gut: *Necrotizing fasciitis* (NF), or flesh-eating disease, is usually caused by more than one type of bacteria and in up to a third of all cases methicillin-resistant *Staphylococcus aureus* (MRSA) is involved. Another bacteria that can cause flesh-eating disease is a certain type of the common bacteria *Streptococci*.

Streptococci is also involved in many conditions from strep throat to pneumonia. The Streptococci family, however, happens to contain friendly types that exist naturally in the gut, and that are commonly used for the production of Swiss cheese!

Ms. Natural: Is malaria caused by a bacteria?

Doc Gut: Malaria is the result of neither a bacteria nor a virus. It's caused by a special type of single-celled microorganism called a parasitic protozoa, which is transmitted by a mosquito. It affects millions of people, resulting in hundred of thousands of deaths every year, mostly in Africa. Although it has dramatically decreased over the last 15 years, malaria is still is one of most serious health problems in the world.

Ms. Natural: How can we avoid being attacked by bad guys?

Doc Gut: There are different approaches. One is to strengthen your immune system to have a better chance of fighting them off. Some alternative health experts recommend exposing children to bacteria and viruses when they are young. Another approach is to try to avoid them as much as possible by being ultra clean, and also by being especially careful when you travel.

The primary preventive measure of modern medicine is vaccinations. Most experts would agree that vaccinations have saved millions of lives. Today there is a great deal of controversy about vaccinations. Some alternative health experts feel these vaccinations can be harmful, especially when several are given at one time to a young child.

REFERENCES:

See Wikipedia for more details on each of each of these microorganisms.

Dutilh, BE et al., Unknown sequences in faecal metagenomes reveal a widely distributed and highly abundant bacteriophage. *Nat. Commun* 2014; 5:4498

Minot, S et al., The human gut virome: Inter-individual variation and dynamic response to diet. *Genome Research* 2011; 21 (10): 1616–1625

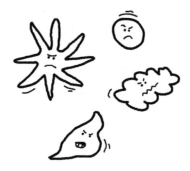

PART 2

DISEASES

CHAPTER 10

Irritable Bowel Syndrome or IBS

I was amazed to learn that the number one digestive disorder in the US is a condition called irritable bowel syndrome or IBS. It affects between 25 and 45 million people of all ages, of which 2 out of 3 are women. If you don't have it, you probably know someone who does.

This disorder can have multiple and sometimes conflicting symptoms, such as an alternation between diarrhea and constipation. You may also have indigestion, excess gas and bloating, or nausea. IBS can be both uncomfortable and debilitating. It is often accompanied by unpredictable abdominal pain, which can be problematic for your social or professional life. The exact cause of this disorder is unknown, but a number of factors contribute to it, including diet, stress, and—guess what?—gut bacteria.

Analysis of stool has revealed that the composition of gut bacteria is different in people suffering from this disorder compared to healthy individuals. Are the different gut bacteria the cause of IBS symptoms or the result? We don't know.

IBS has been treated by probiotics with some success. The most useful probiotics studied include *Lactobacillus plantarum, Bifidobacterium bifidum,* and *Bifidobacterium infantis.* The symptoms that are most consistently relieved by these probiotics are gas and bloating.

One of the most effective natural treatments for IBS is diet. The Low FODMAP Diet, developed by scientists at Monash University in Australia, is the most well-studied. FODMAP lists specific types of food that are poorly absorbed by the upper gut, and which feed gas-producing bacteria in the lower gut.

Why aren't these foods absorbed in the small intestine? There are several reasons. It turns out that about 40% of the population has trouble digesting and absorbing fructose, a condition called fructose malabsorption. (This is not to be confused with hereditary fructose intolerance, which is a far more serious condition caused by a deficiency of certain enzymes in the liver.)

Maybe a piece of cherry pie won't bother us, but when we have it with a soda containing high-fructose corn syrup, things get out of hand. Fructose is not easily absorbed in the small intestine. Instead, it goes down into the colon where it is fermented by the gut bacteria that produce excess gas. Excess gas often results in abdominal pain and bloating, along with either diarrhea or constipation.

Fructose isn't the only culprit. Three-quarters of the world's population have another problem: as they age, they can't digest the same amount of dairy products as they did when they were younger. Milk contains a sugar called lactose, which is split into two simpler sugars by a special enzyme called lactase. Once the splitting occurs, the simple sugars can then be absorbed by the cells in the small intestine.

For some reason, we produce less lactase as we get older, so that the lactose remains undigested in the small intestine, and passes into the large intestine where the gut bacteria ferment it. The result is indigestion and other symptoms of IBS such as excess gas. This doesn't mean that older people can't eat any dairy. It just means that as we age, we need to be much more moderate. We can have some ice cream, we just can't bury it in whipped cream.

Other types of food can cause IBS symptoms. The fiber in most plants is not digested in the small intestine because our digestive system doesn't make the right enzymes to do this. The fiber goes to the large intestine. The bacteria living there possess the right enzymes and can digest the fiber and then ferment it. This, as many have experienced, produces more gas. Fiber is normally considered to be beneficial, but in some people with IBS, it contributes to gas problems.

Gut Rap Q & A:

H Bomb: What exactly does FODMAP stand for?

Doc Gut: The "F" stands for fermentable. "O" stands for oligosaccharides.

H Bomb: Okay, I get the fermentation part. I brew my own beer, so I know the process. But what are oligosaccharides?

Doc Gut: We mentioned them when we talked about breast milk. They are complex sugars, which typically contain 2-10 simple sugar units. Oligosaccharides are not easily digested and pass on to the lower intestine, where they feed the bacteria located there. They occur naturally in certain types of dietary plant fibers.

If we want to be technical, we can classify them into two main types, the fructooligosaccharides (FOS) or fructans, and the galactooligosaccharides (GOS) or galactans. Fructans are present in Jerusalem artichokes, burdock, chicory, leeks, onions, and asparagus. Inulin, a chemical commonly found in processed foods, is one of the main types of fructans or FOS. Galactans, GOS, are naturally found, for example, in soybeans, lentils, and Jerusalem artichokes. They can also be synthesized from lactose (milk sugar) and are frequently used in baby formula.

H Bomb: What about the "D" in FODMAP?

Doc Gut: This "D" stands for disaccharides, which refers to any compound that is composed of 2 simple sugars. For example, sucrose or common sugar is composed of glucose and fructose. Milk sugar, or lactose, is composed of two different sugars, galactose and glucose. In the FODMAP diet, one of the main disaccharides considered is lactose, because, as I mentioned, so many people become lactose intolerant as they get older. (They no longer produce the enzyme lactase that breaks lactose into galactose and glucose. Without this enzyme, lactose goes into the large intestine where it feeds bacteria.)

H Bomb: And the "M"?

Doc Gut: "M" stands for monosaccharides, which are simple sugars like glucose or fructose.

Ms. Natural: Why isn't fructose absorbed easily in the small intestine?

Doc Gut: The cells of the small intestine have special carrier mechanisms for glucose that can easily transport and absorb it into the bloodstream. The carrier mechanism for fructose is different and isn't as effective. If we ingest glucose with fructose, then the fructose is absorbed more easily.

Different types of food have different combinations of glucose and fructose. Bananas are an interesting example. With about twice as much glucose as fructose, they are on the Low FODMAP Diet. Apples have a much higher level of fructose compared to glucose, and as a result, some of the fructose molecules can't get into the cells of the small intestines. They pass instead to the large intestine, where they produce excess gas and cause bloating and distension.

H Bomb: And the "A" and the "P"?

Doc Gut: The "A" just stands for the word "and," so it's really not important.

H Bomb: But they put it in anyway!

Doc Gut: They did. But the "P" stands for polyols. Polyols are sugar alcohols like sorbitol and mannitol, which are commonly added to food to give it a lower caloric content. Some foods, like avocados, naturally contain polyols.

Ms. Natural: How does the diet work?

Doc Gut: Each person reacts differently to these food types, so the Low FODMAP Diet recommends that we go off all gas-producing foods for a month, then gradually re-introduce them one at a time. In this way, we can see the effect of each food on our gut. There are a number of phone apps that can help you with the diet.

Ms. Natural: Is it true that there's a treatment for IBS using essential oils?

Doc Gut: Yes. One significant research finding is that peppermint oil can be beneficial.

H Bomb: I heard about a condition called SIBO. What is it?

Doc Gut: SIBO stands for small intestinal bacterial overgrowth. Normally there are only a few bacteria in the small intestine, but in this condition, there is an overgrowth of bacteria. These bacteria start fermenting the food before it is digested or passed to the lower gut. The result is excess gas, bloating, and burping. There also can be a lack of absorption of valuable nutrients.

The standard treatment for SIBO is antibiotics, but some experts now feel that probiotics should be the first line of treatment, followed by antibiotics only if necessary. Several studies have demonstrated an herbal supplement, as well as specific probiotics, are effective in helping to suppress this bacterial overgrowth in the small intestine.

REFERENCES:

Kennedy, PJ et al., Irritable bowel syndrome: A microbiome-gut-brain axis disorder? *World J Gastroenterol* Oct 2014; 20(39): 14105–14125

The Complete Low-FODMAP Diet: A Revolutionary Plan for Managing IBS and other Digestive Disorders by Sue Shepherd, PhD and Peter Gibson, MD, first published by Penguin, 2011 and then The Experiment, 2013

Brown, K et al., Response of irritable bowel syndrome with constipation patients administered a combined quebracho/conker tree/M. balsamea Willd extract. *World Journal of Gastrointestinal Pharmacology and Therapeutics* 2016; 7(3):463-468

CHAPTER 11

Inflammatory Bowel Disease or IBD

A close friend suffered from inflammatory bowel disease or IBD for many years and was prescribed a variety of medicines, including prednisone. One of the side effects of this corticosteroid drug was that he became permanently blind in one eye. When he was finally operated on, a portion of his large intestine had to be cut away. The surgeon saved the piece of badly ulcerated tissue for him to see. He was shocked to discover that it resembled Swiss cheese.

Over one million people in the US suffer from inflammatory bowel disease. The two main types of IBD are ulcerative colitis (UC) and Crohn's disease. Both conditions cause severe inflammation in the gut lining. UC damages only the colon and rectum, while Crohn's disease can injure any part of the digestive tract.

The exact cause of IBD is unknown, although recent theories suggest a complex interaction between specific factors, including the disruption of the gut bacteria.

According to some scientists, the inception of UC begins in the gut. An abnormal state of gut bacteria aggravates certain immune cells in the gut lining and causes them to produce an exaggerated inflammatory response. Symptoms worsen when infection, antibiotics, diet, drugs, smoking, and stress further agitate these immune cells.

Dysbiosis is the term doctors use to describe an abnormal gut environment. In a state of dysbiosis, the balance between the good and bad bacteria shifts in favor of the bad. Most scientists agree that dysbiosis is significant in the development of IBD.

Studies using germ-free mice are especially convincing as they demonstrate that certain bacteria are necessary for the inception of IBD. Further evidence comes from research that clearly shows that probiotics can improve IBD, especially a probiotic cocktail, which consists of about 17 strains of *Clostridium* (a bacteria that can be either good or bad).

Attempts have been made to understand IBD by analyzing the poop from people who have the disease. The most consistent findings show that IBD patients have a reduced number of bacteria of the phyla *Firmicutes*. Another interesting finding is the presence of an increased concentration of *Escherichia coli,* including pathogenic variants. A new pathogenic group, called adherent-invasive *E. coli* (AIE), has been found in a higher part of the digestive tract in Crohn's patients. The bacteria *Mycobacterium avium paratuberculosis,* or MAP, is also believed to be involved in the development of Crohn's disease.

Some investigators have studied how diet affects IBD. In the case of Crohn's disease, they have used a special diet called exclusive enteral nutrition or EEN—which involves a complete liquid diet for a specific period of time. This diet has been found to induce remission in Crohn's disease, especially in children and adolescents.

Besides probiotics and diet, researchers are studying the effects of fecal transplant for IBD. Results are positive, although somewhat inconsistent. We will have to wait for larger and more carefully controlled studies before probiotics become part of the standard treatment of IBD.

Gut Rap Q & A:

Ms. Natural: What are the symptoms of IBD?

Doc Gut: The most common symptoms are an urgent need to empty the bowels, followed by diarrhea. Some people need to go to the bathroom from 10 to 20 times a day, and are often awakened at night. Another common symptom is stomach pain or cramping. There may also be blood in the stool, fever, fatigue, loss of appetite, and weight loss.

H Bomb: What happens if you have this disease for a long time?

Doc Gut: There are many complications arising from IBD, including fatal colon cancer. But in most cases, diet and drugs manage the disease, though the patient's quality of life may be severely compromised. Because the gut is inflamed, nutrients are not absorbed properly, so special diets and supplements are often necessary. Anemia is another problem, due to the blood loss during elimination. Children can also have growth delays and decreased bone mineral density, not only as a result of IBD, but also due to medications. In Crohn's disease, the formation of scar tissue causes a narrowing of the intestinal walls with further complications.

Ms. Natural: Should someone with this condition be on a specific diet?

Doc Gut: There are so many variations in symptoms that it's hard to say which diet is best for each person. Many experts now recommend some type of special gut repair diet, which will allow the gut to restore itself while providing adequate nutrients.

We highly recommend that anyone experiencing IBS check with a qualified doctor, and also keep a food journal to find out which foods are easiest for them to digest. Every single thing we eat affects our gut bacteria, so it's critical to create a balanced state.

REFERENCES:

Ahmed, I et al., Microbiome, Metabolome and Inflammatory Bowel Disease. *Microorganisms* 2016; 4, 20

Narushima, S et al., Characterization of the 17 strains of regulatory T cell-inducing human-derived Clostridia. *Gut Microbes* May/June 2014; 5:3, 333–339

Konig, J et al., Consensus report: faecal microbiota transfer – clinical applications and procedures. *Aliment Pharmacol Ther* 2017; 45: 222–239

Chu, ND et al., Profiling Living Bacteria Informs Preparation of Fecal Microbiota Transplantations. Zoetendal EG, ed. *PLoS ONE* 2017; 12(1):e0170922

Vermeire, SJ et al., Donor species richness determines faecal microbiota transplantation success in inflammatory bowel disease. *J Crohns Colitis* 2016; 10: 387–94

Van Nood, E et al., Duodenal infusion of donor feces for recurrent Clostridium difficile. *N Engl J Med* 2013; 368(5): 407–15

CHAPTER 12

Brain Wiring

I have spent much of my life studying how experience changes our brain, but I never realized that one of the most influential experiences is the activity of our gut bacteria. Our brain is incredibly dynamic. Everything we do, everything we see, everything we feel, changes its wiring. And our brain is especially flexible and sensitive when we are young. Studies show that the quality of the early environment can even determine the number of connections in the brain and its chemical makeup. It has only recently been discovered, however, how important the state of the digestive system is to the wiring of the human brain.

In her book, *Gut and Psychology Syndrome*, Dr. Natasha Campbell-McBride states that in her clinical experience she has yet to meet a child with autism, hyperactivity, inability to learn, or mood and behavioral disorders, who does not have some gut abnormalities. The digestive system, she states, holds the key to a child's mental development. Other doctors and scientists have also made this important observation.

Most of the autistic children she treats in her clinic develop fussy eating habits early in their lives. They end up with a very limited diet, which includes only a few food groups, often sweet and starchy. These children tend to have diarrhea or constipation, as well as flatulence and bloating. Autistic children have difficulty communicating, so these symptoms can go unnoticed or untreated. As she explains, it was not until about 20 years ago that doctors first started to research the connection between autism and gut problems. What they noticed at the time were inflamed lymph nodes in parts of the gut wall resembling ulcerative colitis. Comprehensive studies have now documented the widespread occurrence of digestive disorders in autistic patients.

In 2013, it was estimated that Autism Spectrum Disorder or ASD affects over 20 million people, and this number keeps growing. It is present in boys about five times more often than girls. ASD affects how the brain processes information, and its main symptoms include difficulty in social interactions, language impairment, and repetitive behavior.

Despite the writing of Dr. Campbell-McBride and others, the evidence that ASD is caused or influenced by diet or abnormal gut bacteria is still controversial. Most scientists believe that ASD is the result of genetic and environmental influences. There are many animal studies, however, that strongly implicate gut bacteria as an important factor.

In one animal model, autistic-like behavior was induced by injecting pregnant mice with an immune system stimulant. Babies born from these abnormal mothers displayed several autistic characteristics. They had peculiar social interactions, spent less time in an open space, had repetitive behavior, were more easily startled by sounds, and produced fewer vocalizations. They also had gut disorders. When the bacteria *Bacteroides fragilis* was given to these mice, their gut problems and autistic-like behavior went away.

In another study, female mice were given a high-fat diet in order to induce autistic behavior in the offspring. When the over-fed mothers bred and bore offspring, the babies showed behavioral traits similar to autism, spending less time with other mice and displaying abnormal social interactions. Investigators then looked at the composition of the gut bacteria, and found clear differences in those fed a high-fat diet compared to healthy mother mice.

The researchers looked at several ways by which the babies might be cured of the autistic symptoms. First, they put the autistic baby mice in with other normal mice. Typically, mice eat each other's poop—a common practice among some animals, called coprophagia, which we have mentioned before. When the autistic mice ate the poop of the healthy mice, it acted like an oral fecal transplant and their behavior became normal.

Second, the researchers gave the autistic mice the probiotic *Lactobacillus reuteri*. (You may remember that *L. reuteri* is one of the good bacteria.) When the mice consumed this bacteria, several important aspects of their social behavior became normal. It was also found that *L. reuteri* increased the production of oxytocin, the "bonding hormone," as well as restoring abnormal changes in reward centers of the brains of these mice.

In one study on humans, the species *Lactobacillus plantarum* was given to children with Autistic Syndrome Disorder. Half of these children were randomly given the probiotic and half were given a placebo. The parents of the children taking the probiotic noticed many positive results, and decided that the happiness of their children was more important than the study. These parents refused to switch their children to the placebo group, and the study had to be discontinued because there were simply not enough control subjects.

The data is not all in on other neurological disorders, but initial results are provocative. Consider Parkinson's disease. Like autism, it has been noted for many years that patients with Parkinson's have constipation and other digestive problems. In many cases, digestive problems have been reported from up to 10 years before the actual onset of symptoms of the disease. Studies show that people with Parkinson's have a different composition of gut bacteria from that of healthy adults. When a group of researchers placed gut bacteria from human Parkinson's patients into germ-free mice, the animals quickly deteriorated with Parkinson-like symptoms.

In the case of Alzheimer's sufferers, gut bacteria have also been implicated. Recent studies show that the gut bacteria can cause the blood-brain barrier to become more permeable to unwanted substances, such as microbes. This could lead to the following sequence of events: increased risk of infection, activation of the brain's immune system, and the resulting deposit of beta-amyloid plaque found in the brains of Alzheimer's patients. One study also has shown that intestinal bacteria can accelerate the development of Alzheimer's disease in mice. Intestinal bacteria was transferred from diseased mice to germ-free mice, with the result that the mice developed more beta-amyloid plaques in the brain compared to controls.

Many experts consider multiple sclerosis or MS to be an auto-immune disease. In MS, immune cells attack the fatty sheath or myelin that covers and protects nerve fibers. Myelin allows nerve cells to transmit information at a high speed. When it is destroyed, the nervous system can't function properly, leading to many debilitating physical and mental symptoms.

In studies on mice with an MS-like disease, it has been shown that altering the gut microbiome produces changes in the immune system and reduces symptoms of the disease. Mice were also prevented from getting the MS-like disease in the first place by receiving a gut-related molecule called polysaccharide A. Exploratory human studies demonstrate that patients with MS have a different composition of gut bacteria, with fewer good bacteria. These studies, as well as others, have led some scientists to suggest that altering gut bacteria may be a cure for MS and other autoimmune diseases that affect the brain.

Gut Rap Q & A

Ms. Natural: What causes autism?

Doc Gut: No one knows for sure. Initial signs are typically noticed in the first two years of life. Autism is often inherited, so genetic factors are considered to be important. Environmental factors have also been implicated. For example, one of the most controversial factors, which we mentioned before, is the injection of multiple vaccines at an early age.

Ms. Natural: How does autism affect the brain?

Doc Gut: It influences neural development and how the brain processes information. One of the most important areas in the brain disturbed is the prefrontal cortex and an interesting study suggests that the gut bacteria play a significant role in the regulation of certain genes involved in the neural development of the prefrontal cortex. Autistic children tend to have higher levels of inflammation in the brain, and this could be another connection with gut bacteria.

Ms. Natural: I have heard that the number of people being diagnosed with it is increasing.

Doc Gut: Yes, that is true. The number has increased dramatically, with a 30% increase from 2012 to 2014 in the US. We don't know if this increase is due to changes in diagnostic practice or changes in other factors such as gut bacteria.

Ms. Natural: Why is it now called Autistic Spectrum Disorder?

Doc Gut: There are different types of autistic disorders, which have been grouped under the general heading of Autism Spectrum Disorder. People with this disorder display symptoms in their own unique manner. Some have remarkable skills and intellectual abilities, and through various treatment programs are able to function independently in the world. One of the most notable examples is author, speaker, and autism expert Temple Grandin.

Almost one-third of people who have ASD communicate nonverbally. To understand more about this condition, we recommend an inspiring and informative YouTube video called "In My Language."

H Bomb: I read something about a substance called EPS that might be the cause of autism.

Doc Gut: You're getting up-to-date on the research, aren't you?

H Bomb: I try to keep up.

Doc Gut: Caltech researchers found EPS (4-ethylphenyl sulfate) in the serum of autistic-like mice. The autistic mice had 46 times more EPS than healthy mice. EPS is similar to a substance in the urine of autistic children.

When autistic mice were treated with *B. fragilis*, their EPS levels returned to normal. It is thought that by repairing the leaky guts of these mice, the *B. fragilis* bacteria had probably stopped the EPS from getting into the brain and causing the autistic behavior.

Ms. Natural: Wasn't epilepsy once treated with diet?

Doc Gut: That's true. In the 1920s, epilepsy was treated with a diet developed at the Mayo Clinic called the "ketogenic diet." This diet restricted carbohydrates and proteins, replacing them with fats. The results were so successful that the medical community commonly used this diet until 1938 when anti-epileptic and anticonvulsant drugs were introduced, and doctors felt the drugs were more effective. But many would argue today that this diet has far fewer side effects.

REFERENCES:

Gut and Psychology Syndrome by Dr. Natasha Campbell-McBride, MD, Medinform Publishing Cambridge, UK, 2010

Chaidez, V et al., Gastrointestinal problems in children with autism, developmental delays or typical development. *Journal of autism and developmental disorders.* 2014; 44(5):1117-1127

Krajmalnik-Brown, R et al., Gut bacteria in children with autism spectrum disorders: challenges and promise of studying how a complex community influences a complex disease. *Microbial Ecology in Health and Disease* 2015; 26:10.3402/mehd.v26.26914

Hsiao, EY et al., Microbiota modulate behavioral and physiological abnormalities associated with neurodevelopmental disorders. *Cell* 2013; 155:1451–63

Buffington, SA, et al., Microbial Reconstitution Reverses Maternal Diet-Induced Social and Synaptic Deficits in Offspring. *Cell* Jun 2016; 165(7):1762-75

Parracho, H et al., A Double-Blind, Placebo-Controlled, Crossover-Designed Probiotic Feeding Study In Children Diagnosed With Autistic Spectrum Disorders, *International Journal of Probiotics and Prebiotics* 2010; 5, 2, 69-74

Braniste, VA et al., The gut microbiota influences blood-brain barrier permeability in mice. *Science translational medicine.* 2014; 6(263):263ra158

Harach, T et al., Reduction of Abeta amyloid pathology in APPPS1 transgenic mice in the absence of gut microbiota. *Scientific Reports*, 2017; 7: 41802 DOI: 10.1038/srep41802

"In My Language." (*https://www.youtube.com/ watch?v=JnylM1hI2jc*)

CHAPTER 13

Heart Matters

Heart disease is the number one killer in the world, and at some point most of us feel vulnerable, for either ourselves or a loved one.

Gut bacteria play a role in heart disease and the risk factors associated with it. We have already mentioned one of the major risk factors for heart disease, obesity. Research shows that gut bacteria are involved in obesity, and ongoing research will reveal if changing the gut bacteria can help cure this condition.

Another important risk factor is high blood pressure, which affects over 1 billion people around the world. In an extraordinary study done by Dr. Jennifer L. Pluznick and her team at the Johns Hopkins University School of Medicine, gut bacteria were shown to produce substances that influence the kidney to help lower blood pressure.

Let me explain her very interesting research: First, odor-sensing receptors, typically located in the nose, have been found in the walls of small blood vessels in many different organs throughout the body, including the kidney, heart, diaphragm, skeletal muscles, and skin.

Second, the short-chain fatty acids (SCFAs) produced by gut bacteria enter the bloodstream and interact with these odor-sensing receptors.

Third, once the SCFAs interact with the receptors, the results, although complex, show an overall lowering of blood pressure.

Other animal studies and human clinical trials demonstrate that changes in gut bacteria can improve blood pressure, either through probiotics or diet. The mechanisms of how this is done are still under investigation.

Another risk factor is high cholesterol. In one study on 900 subjects in the Netherlands, it was found that gut bacteria are strongly linked to healthy levels of good cholesterol (HDL) and triglycerides. The researchers concluded that altering gut bacteria might be a new means to improve blood cholesterol levels.

A further risk factor for heart disease is diabetes. Preliminary research shows a relationship between the composition of the gut bacteria and diabetes. There are two main types of diabetes: types 1 and 2. In both conditions, the patient is unable to regulate blood sugar (glucose) levels, which can lead to serious health problems.

Type 1 is considered an autoimmune disease in which our own immune system destroys special cells in the pancreas that make insulin. Insulin allows glucose to move from the bloodstream into the cells of the body. There have been speculations that type 1 diabetes, like other autoimmune diseases, may be caused by an abnormal condition in the gut.

Type 2 is far more common and is caused by an inability of the body to use the insulin (insulin resistance). Many animal studies find a correlation between diabetes markers and gut bacteria, and there are detailed theories of how an abnormal state of gut bacteria can lead to inflammation, which in turn leads to the inability to regulate glucose levels. One study in Russia analyzed the composition of the gut bacteria and blood glucose levels in approximately 90 patients who had either diabetes or prediabetes, or who were healthy. Researchers were able to link the inability to maintain normal glucose levels with specific types of bacteria. Clinical trials are currently being done in the US to test the efficacy of probiotics in helping to improve type 2 diabetes.

In addition to these studies, other research has shown that patients with heart disease have a different composition of gut bacteria from that of normal subjects. Many doctors and scientists now feel that one of the most crucial factors in the development of heart disease is chronic inflammation, particularly in the lining of arteries around the heart. And gut bacteria have clearly been implicated in an increase in the inflammatory response, particularly in the gut. If it can be shown that an abnormal state of gut bacteria overexcites specific immune cells in the coronary arteries, this will further reveal a link between disrupted gut bacteria and the development of heart disease.

Gut Rap Q & A:

Ms. Natural: Aren't there bacteria that can damage the heart?

Doc Gut: There are. The best example is the *Streptococcus* bacteria. This bacteria commonly causes strep throat, which can lead to rheumatic fever and the rarer scarlet fever. These are both inflammatory disorders that can result in damage to the heart valves. Rheumatic fever occurs in about 325,000 children each year worldwide, and about 18 million people currently have rheumatic heart disease, especially in developing countries.

The *Streptococcus* bacteria has resulted in the widespread use and misuse of antibiotics. Doctors who saw a child with what they believed to be strep throat would prescribe an antibiotic to avoid the rare chance of rheumatic fever, which was greatly feared because of its lifelong damaging effects to the heart. This can be avoided by doing a simple throat culture to test for the bacteria before giving the antibiotics.

H Bomb: Is smoking a cardiovascular risk factor?

Doc Gut: Yes, it is, and we talked in a previous chapter about how gut bacteria are affected by smoking.

H Bomb: What about metabolic syndrome?

Doc Gut: Metabolic syndrome is the combination of a number of risk factors we have discussed, such as obesity, high blood pressure, abnormal cholesterol levels, and diabetes or prediabetes.

Evidence strongly suggests that altering bacteria can improve metabolic syndrome.

Ms. Natural: What are the effects of probiotics on heart disease?

Doc Gut: We see promising results in animal studies. Using specific types of probiotics, there have been reductions in both obesity and diabetes, and improvements in key biochemical measures. Human studies will give a clearer idea of how to use probiotics and diet to change the composition of the gut bacteria and help both prevent and treat heart disease.

REFERENCES:

Pluznick, JL et al., Olfactory receptor responding to gut microbiota-derived signals plays a role in renin secretion and blood pressure regulation *PNAS* 2013 110 (11) 4410-4415

de Brito Alves, JL et al., New Insights on the Use of Dietary Polyphenols or Probiotics for the Management of Arterial Hypertension. *Front. Physiol* 2016; 7:448

Robles-Vera, I et al., Antihypertensive Effects of Probiotics. Curr Hypertens Rep. Apr 2017;19(4):26

Fu, J et al., The Gut Microbiome Contributes to a Substantial Proportion of the Variation in Blood Lipids. *Circulation Research* 2015; 117:817-824

Musso, G et al., Obesity, Diabetes, and Gut Microbiota: The hygiene hypothesis expanded? *Diabetes Care* 2010; 33(10):2277-2284

Tuovinen, E et al., Cytokine response of human mononuclear cells induced by intestinal Clostridium species. *Anaerobe* 2013; 19(1)

Marijon, E et al., Rheumatic heart disease. *Lancet* 2012; 379 (9819): 953–64

Festi, D et al., Gut microbiota and metabolic syndrome. *World J Gastroenterol* November 2014; 21; 20(43): 16079-16094

CHAPTER 14

Gut Imbalance Equals Dis-ease

In researching this book we were amazed to see how many human diseases might be caused or aggravated by an abnormal state of the gut bacteria. We have already mentioned many of the most important diseases, but it is useful to consider a few more interesting examples.

Two diseases that have been studied intensively are asthma and allergies. Numerous studies, as we mentioned, have shown a strong correlation between babies born with a caesarean birth and the development of childhood asthma and allergies. We have also seen studies showing that the composition of an infant's gut bacteria is very different depending on the birth method.

In a large study in Denmark, the records of almost 2 million children were examined over a 35-year period and a strong correlation was found between caesarean birth and asthma, as well as other conditions. This means that the risk of developing asthma after a caesarean birth is 20% higher than a normal birth. While other factors such as genetics and air pollution play a role, many researchers now feel that the lack of introduction of certain friendly gut bacteria with caesarean birth is an important cause of the recent increase in asthma and allergies.

Another interesting finding is that gut bacteria may influence the severity of a stroke, which is the second leading cause of death worldwide. Two groups of mice were studied, each with a different composition of gut bacteria. A stroke was induced in both groups and brain damage was measured. In Group 1, the brain damage was 60% less than Group 2. The gut bacteria in Group 1 caused an increase in a beneficial type of immune cell, which helped lessen the effects of the stroke. The gut bacteria in Group 2 caused an increase in a different type of immune cells, which produced a chemical that can cause harmful inflammation after the stroke. Researchers felt that the results of this study could eventually lead to a new procedure for the prevention of strokes in high-risk patients by altering gut bacteria.

Finally, we come to the relationship between cancer and gut bacteria, which my friend had been skeptical about. Animal studies have determined that certain beneficial bacteria can help to delay and slow down the onset of cancer in cells of the immune system. Mice with these particular good bacteria lived four times longer and had less DNA damage and inflammation. Gut bacteria have also been found to improve the use of one anti-cancer drug in animals with cancer, making it twice as effective at reducing tumors.

Gut Rap Q & A:

Ms. Natural: Do you think probiotics will someday cure all disease?

H Bomb: Come ON. I suppose they're also going to help my missing leg grow back.

Ms. Natural: Oh, I'm so sorry, I didn't realize that you were missing a leg.

H Bomb: I was speaking *metaphorically*.

Doc Gut: Let's get back to Ms. Natural's original question. We have no idea yet if probiotics will cure all diseases. There are many probiotic treatments that work in animals, but not in humans. Everyone is excited about the possibilities of probiotics, but it will take a great deal more research to answer your question.

Ms. Natural: When will this research be done?

Doc Gut: It's hard to say. Remember earlier that we had mentioned over 1000 clinical trials are going on for all different types of dis-ease. And because of the success of fecal transplants for *C. difficile,* there are over 100 clinical trials on the use of fecal transplants for different conditions. But even these studies will probably not be enough since the ecology of the gut bacteria is so complex, and so many different possible types of probiotics need to be studied.

H Bomb: Who participates in such trials?

Doc Gut: People who are sick. If you have ulcerative colitis or some other serious condition, you might be willing to try anything. There are even websites that promote doing a home made fecal transplant under a doctor's supervision. There are many disorders that Western medicine has not been able to treat and the drugs used can produce unpleasant side effects, so many people have turned to alternative health practices.

REFERENCES:

Sevelsted, A et al., Cesarean Section and Chronic Immune Disorders. *Pediatrics* January 2015; 135,1

Brandão, HV et al., Increased risk of allergic rhinitis among children delivered by cesarean section: a cross-sectional study nested in a birth cohort. *BMC Pediatrics* 2016; 16:57

Houghteling, PD and Walker, WA, From birth to "immuno-health", allergies and enterocolitis. *Journal of clinical gastroenterology* 2015; 49(0 1):S7-S12

Campbell, AW, Autoimmunity and the Gut. *Autoimmune Diseases* 2014; 2014:152428

Benakis, C et al., Commensal microbiota affects ischemic stroke outcome by regulating intestinal γδ T cells. *Nature Medicine*, 2016; 22(5):516-23

For information on clinical trials go to: https://clinicaltrials.gov/ and enter "fecal microbiome transplant" and "probiotics" in the search box.

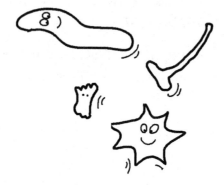

PART 3

HOW DOES OUR GUT WORK?

CHAPTER 15

The Gut Barrier

As I watched *Lord of the Rings* for probably the 22nd time, the final battle made me think of the human gut. The fortress at the capital of Gondor and our gut both have outer and inner walls to repel enemies and prevent them from taking over. In both cases, if the outer wall is breached, there are several inner walls, with more warriors ready to continue the fight.

In an adult, the gut barrier runs from mouth to anus (30 feet long) with a defense system consisting of multiple outer and inner walls that exclude microbes and unwanted substances from entering our "inner body."

The innermost wall of the gut barrier is the most vulnerable and is constantly under attack from bacteria inside the gut. Anatomists call this wall the mucosa or mucosal layer. It contains three or four inner walls or sublayers. The first sublayer of the mucosal wall is a coating of mucus secreted by cells in the gut lining. Containing special proteins called mucins, which have an antimicrobial effect, we might compare the mucus to the moat of a castle filled with protective magical beasts.

The second sublayer is the gut lining, with cells that are tightly bound together in a column-like organization. This sublayer selectively allows water and nutrients to cross the cell membranes and enter the bloodstream. It also keeps bacteria and toxins out. We can compare it to the gated main wall of a castle, with guards who only allow certain people inside.

The third sublayer is the lamina propria. It contains blood vessels, nerves, and most importantly, immune cells—the troops of the gut barrier. The lamina propria is like an area behind the main wall of the castle where soldiers stand ready for a first wave of attack. The fourth sublayer is a thin lining of smooth muscle cells that keep the cells and glands in a constant state of gentle agitation.

Beneath the mucosa wall is the submucosal wall or layer. It is the second major wall, and within it are a vast collection of specialized cells including glands, blood vessels, muscles, nerve cells, and more immune cells. This submucosal wall acts as a secondary line of defense to deal with any bacteria that might get through the first four sublayers of the mucosa wall.

Beyond this defense system are two thicker layers, which serve a different purpose. The first of these is the muscular layer, which contains smooth muscles and is responsible for the movement of food through the GI tract. Next is the serosa, which is made of connective tissue and separates the gut from other tissues in the body.

The gut's own immune system, as we have mentioned, is called the gut-associated lymphatic tissue or GALT. It contains a high percentage of all the cells in the body's immune system and includes many different types of immune cells, such as macrophages, B cells, and T cells. All of these immune cells work together to help terminate foreign invaders.

The GALT defense system has a series of small "forts" along the gut barrier. These "forts," called Peyer's patches, are loaded with lymph tissue and immune cells, and are located right next to the cell lining of the mucosal wall. In the gut lining are M cells (microfold cells), which act as "scouts" to identify and "interrogate" harmful bacteria. As a result, immune cells are alerted throughout the body to any potential enemy. Some bad bacteria are immediately destroyed or engulfed by the gut immune cells. Others are identified, marked for destruction, and eliminated in a massive battle, which employs lethal biochemical warfare secreted by different types of immune cells.

These are only a few of the unique features of our gut barrier. The specific characteristics of the gut walls change depending on the needs of that particular part of the GI tract. One way that good bacteria help is through a process called colonization resistance, in which beneficial bacteria protect us simply by occupying space along the mucus sublayer that would otherwise be taken by bad bacteria (possession being 9/10 of the law).

This is a sophisticated and highly efficient border wall. Donald Trump would be impressed.

Gut Rap Q & A:

Ms. Natural: Can you explain again why friendly gut bacteria are important to a healthy gut barrier?

Doc Gut: One of the most important activities of our gut bacteria is the development of the gut walls and some of the immune cells in it. At an early age, the types of bacteria present in the gut educate the immune cells about good and bad bacteria. This can be seen clearly in germ-free mice. Without the presence of gut bacteria, the immune cells in their gut wall do not develop properly, but the problem can be remedied with the introduction of friendly bacteria.

H Bomb: How do bad bacteria breach the gut barrier?

Doc Gut: Take cholera as an example. It is caused by the bacteria *Vibrio cholera* and results in a huge loss of bodily fluids. The bacteria penetrates the acid environment of the stomach and lodges itself in the walls of the small intestine. There it produces toxins that cause excessive amounts of water to move from inside the body to the gut, leading to severe diarrhea and even death.

Some bacteria, such as *Salmonella* and *Shigella,* can trick certain defending cells in the gut barrier to engulf them. When this is done, these bacteria have the ability to reverse engineer the engulfing process and escape. Other bacteria use different forms of chemical warfare, for example, secreting enzymes to penetrate the cells lining the gut and cause damage inside.

REFERENCES:

Groschwitz, KR and Hogan, SP, Intestinal Barrier Function: Molecular Regulation and Disease Pathogenesis. *The Journal of allergy and clinical immunology* 2009; 124(1):3-22

Bischoff, SC et al., Intestinal permeability – a new target for disease prevention and therapy. *BMC Gastroenterology* 2014; 14:189

Viggiano, D et al., Gut barrier in health and disease: focus on child-hood. *Eur Rev Med Pharmacol Sci* 2015; 19, 6, 1077-1085

See also GALT, Peyer's patch, and microfold or M cells in Wikipedia.

CHAPTER 16

The Gut-Brain Axis

Most people are not aware that they have a "second nervous system" inside their gut, which can operate independently of the central and peripheral nervous systems. This gut nervous system is called the enteric nervous system (ENS) and consists of 500 million nerve cells—fewer than the brain's nearly 100 billion nerve cells, but comparable to the entire central nervous system of a small mammal. The ENS communicates with our brain via nerves and chemical messengers. A stressed brain, for example, triggers a cascade of nerve impulses and hormones that signal the ENS to shut down the digestive process.

The ENS monitors and regulates the gut, sending signals to our brain that identify every detail of digestion, such as gut mobility, chemicals in the digestive tract, and the level of acidity. Some gut functions are regulated locally, such as the movement of food in the gut or immune cell functions in the gut wall, but other activities, such as appetite and overall digestion, are controlled through the gut-brain axis. The gut-brain axis consists of all the complex interactions between the brain, ENS, immune system, endocrine system, and the gut bacteria.

Let's consider a few types of communication in the gut-brain axis. The most direct is through the vagus nerve, an important and long nerve in the body, which regulates many internal functions. The vagus nerve starts in the brain and branches to the throat, heart, lungs, digestive system, and other parts of the body. It transports messages directly from the brain to the gut, and from the gut to the brain.

A less direct means of communication is through different chemical messengers, such as neurotransmitters and hormones. Each part of the gut-brain axis does this differently. Our main nervous system, for example, sends out nerve impulse signals to all parts of the body, which can release neurotransmitters to activate muscles and other nerve cells. The endocrine system secretes hormones that go through the bloodstream to many parts of the body including the gut. When a harmful bacteria comes into contact with a certain type of immune cell, the cell releases numerous chemical messengers such as cytokines, which activate other immune cells in the area and throughout the body. The ENS produces more than 30 neurotransmitters, which are exactly the same as the neurotransmitters in the brain. In fact, the gut produces a larger quantity of neurotransmitters than the brain.

We now know that gut bacteria can produce their own vast array of chemical messengers that go into the bloodstream and act on cells in the brain and body. In this way, messages can go from our brain to the gut, from the gut to our brain, and among all of the systems involved. Our knowledge of the gut-brain axis is constantly growing and will contribute to a deeper understanding of the gut's profound influence on the health of our body and mind.

Gut Rap Q & A:

H Bomb: What types of neurotransmitters does the ENS make?

Doc Gut: One example is the mood-altering neurotransmitter serotonin. More than 90% of the body's serotonin is formed in the gut. Another example is dopamine, a neurotransmitter often associated with addiction. The gut produces about 50% of the body's dopamine.

H Bomb: Do gut bacteria produce neurotransmitters?

Doc Gut: Yes, they do. One of the first to be discovered was the neurotransmitter gamma-aminobutyric acid (GABA). This molecule is a major inhibitory neurotransmitter in the central and enteric nervous systems.

Ms. Natural: How do the immune system and nervous system work together?

Doc Gut: We know that if we interpret an event as stressful, our nervous system reacts. One of the main stress centers in our brain is the amygdala. When anything stressful happens to us, a reaction begins in the amygdala and then continues on to other areas of the body, including our autonomic nervous system, endocrine system, digestive system, and immune system.

We go into a fight-or-flight response, during which our digestive system effectively shuts down. Our adrenal glands produce the stress hormone cortisol, which dampens the activity of our immune system. Every psychological state we experience has a corresponding physiological state, which involves the interaction of all of these systems. What is new is that we now recognize that the gut bacteria are part of this important network.

REFERENCES:

Carabotti, M et al., The gut-brain axis: interactions between enteric microbiota, central and enteric nervous systems. *Annals of Gastroenterology* 2015; 28, 203-209

Mu, C et al., Gut Microbiota: The Brain Peacekeeper. *Frontiers in Microbiology.* March 2016; 7, 345

Konturek, PC et al., Stress and the gut: pathophysiology, clinical consequences, diagnostic approach and treatment options. *J Physiol Pharmacol* Dec 2011; 62(6):591-9

CHAPTER 17

Leaky Gut Syndrome

The term "Leaky Gut Syndrome" is commonly used on the Internet and in magazine articles to refer to a range of digestive symptoms, including gas, bloating, cramps, nausea, indigestion, heartburn, and food sensitivity. Conservative doctors do not like the term Leaky Gut Syndrome, calling it a very gray area, a medical mystery, and not a term you find in medical textbooks. Even Wikipedia gives it a slap in the face, defining it as a hypothetical, medically unrecognized condition.

It's not new for doctors and alternative health experts to disagree. This issue, however, is especially confusing. Everyone understands that the gut lining is a critical barrier, which keeps out anything that might be dangerous to the body. It does, however, allow digested food substances to cross the cell membranes of the absorptive cells lining the gut, which includes amino acids, simple sugars, and fatty acids, as well as specific vitamins and minerals. From the absorptive cells, the food particles are then moved into the bloodstream or lymph system. The liver and other tissues eventually process the food particles for energy use, storage, and structure.

Food particles, however, do not normally enter the body through the junctions between the cells. Tight junctions close off the spaces between the absorptive cells. In certain disorders and infections, however, an abnormal situation occurs in which these tight junctions open, allowing undigested food and various substances to leak through. Doctors refer to this situation as "increased intestinal permeability."

If this is the case, why doesn't the medical establishment like the term Leaky Gut Syndrome? Isn't it the same as increased intestinal permeability? I believe the real disagreement comes from the use of the expression leaky gut by so many alternative health experts to promote unproven treatments and commercial products to correct the syndrome. Most doctors know that such recommendations haven't been properly researched.

There are clear exceptions. Celiac disease, for example, is a well-studied genetic disorder in which the tight junctions of the gut wall are disrupted by the gluten in wheat and other foods. In celiac disease, the junctions between the cells loosen and the integrity of the wall is lost. This allows gliadin, a component of gluten, to get through the wall, and causes an immediate immune response. The result is excessive inflammation, which damages vital cells and hampers the absorption of nutrients, eventually leading to an incurable autoimmune disease and a lifetime intolerance to wheat, barley, rye, and other grains that contain or are contaminated by gluten. Surely, this should be a valid example of a leaky gut!

Medical experts say "no," and continue to refer to celiac as an increase in intestinal permeability. The debate goes on. What is clear is that the gut bacteria play a vital role in ensuring that gut walls remain tightly sealed. Whether we subscribe to the term Leaky Gut Syndrome or intestinal permeability, our gut bacteria and diet are indisputably key players in both conditions.

Gut Rap Q & A:

H Bomb: Why don't they just stop fighting and do the research?

Doc Gut: Good point. Medical experts want carefully controlled human studies, which cost a great deal of money. They don't like it when the alternative health experts say they can cure everything with probiotics, supplements, and diet. Yet all the research suggests that these may well be the best solutions to many of today's health problems.

Ms. Natural: Can you tell us a little more about how the tight junctions in our gut become leaky?

Doc Gut: Tight junctions are created by structural proteins (such as claudin and occludin), which span two adjoining cells and bind them together. Zonulin is a regulatory protein in the small intestines that can control the seal of tight junctions. Patients with celiac disease produce more zonulin, which causes the tight junctions to become loose. This increases intestinal permeability to the point where larger food particles, such as gliadin, can penetrate between two adjoining cells and directly enter the bloodstream.

H Bomb: How does this zonulin thing work?

Doc Gut: There are tiny receptors on the surface of the cells that line the small intestines that are sensitive to gliadin. Celiac patients have more of these receptors than other people. When the gliadin molecules come into contact with these receptors they fit into them like a key in a lock and this causes the production of zonulin, which then opens the tight junctions and allows the gliadin to get into the bloodstream where it provokes an immune response.

The cholera bacteria *Vibrio cholera*, as we mentioned, also has the ability to open the tight junctions. It releases a toxin that fits into these cell receptors and also causes an increased production of zonulin. The cells come apart and fluids from the inside of the body pour into the gut resulting in diarrhea. This massive loss of fluids can be fatal.

H Bomb: Can bacteria interact with tight junctions?

Doc Gut: There is new research that suggests that certain bacteria can affect tight junctions in the large intestine using a mechanism, which is different from zonulin.

Ms. Natural: How does food normally get from inside the gut to the rest of our body? Is it through these junctions?

Doc Gut: No, as we mentioned, food particles don't normally pass between cells of the gut lining. They go across the cell membranes so that the food particles are properly digested before they enter the bloodstream.

H Bomb: How does that work again?

Doc Gut: Food is digested into its smallest components by enzymes that are secreted into the gut by the mouth, stomach, pancreas, and small intestine. Once the food has been broken down by the enzymes and others on the surface of the cells lining the gut, the smaller food particles are then transported across the membranes of the cells in the small intestine. These absorptive cells that line the gut, enterocytes, have special folds called microvilli, which greatly expand the surface area of the membrane. If you were to calculate the total area of all the cell membranes, it would be the size of about half a badminton court.

Ms. Natural: How do the foods get transported into the cell?

Doc Gut: Most food substances must be actively carried across the membranes by special transport or carrier mechanisms. These membrane transporters are particular for each type of food. There is a glucose transporter, an amino acid transporter, a free fatty acid transporter, etc. Once the food particles are inside the cell, they are then moved by similar mechanisms into the bloodstream for metabolism in the liver and other parts of the body. Fats are unique in that they go from cells in the small intestine directly to the lymph system, and then into the bloodstream.

Ms. Natural: What does the gallbladder do?

Doc Gut: Our gallbladder assists the digestion of fats by storing and releasing bile, which helps to emulsify fats so they are more easily digested in the small intestine.

Ms. Natural: Is gluten the main problem in Leaky Gut Syndrome?

Doc Gut: Most alternative health experts would agree that gluten is the culprit, but some include all grains. The reason is that most grains have substances similar to gluten that are hard to digest.

H Bomb: What are these substances?

Doc Gut: One of these substances is a special storage protein called prolamin. Gluten contains a prolamin called gliadin. Prolamins are found in many other grains as well, such as: barley (hordein), rye (secalin), corn (zein), sorghum (kafirin), oats (avenin), and rice (orzenin). Another type of substance in grains that is difficult to digest is lectin, which we will talk more about later.

REFERENCES:

Sturgeon, C and Fasano, A, Zonulin, a regulator of epithelial and endothelial barrier functions, and its involvement in chronic inflammatory diseases. *Tissue Barriers* 2016; 4(4):e1251384

Arrieta, MC et al., Alterations in intestinal permeability. *Gut* 2006; 55(10):1512-1520

Kong, W et al., Effect of Bacillus subtilis on Aeromonas hydrophila-induced intestinal mucosal barrier function damage and inflammation in grass carp (Ctenopharyngodon idella). *Scientific Reports* 2017; 7:1588

Chelakkot, C et al., Intestinal Epithelial Cell-Specific Deletion of PLD2 Alleviates DSS-Induced Colitis by Regulating Occludin. *Scientific Reports* 2017; 7:1573

Sipola, S et al., Colon epithelial injury in critically ill colectomized patients: aberration of tight junction proteins and Toll-like receptors. *Minerva Anestesiol* 2017 Apr 13

Helander, HF and Fändriks L, Surface area of the digestive tract - revisited. *Scand J Gastroenterol* 2014; 49(6):681-9

CHAPTER 18

Appetite

Is it my gut bacteria who are craving chocolate ice cream, or is it me? Wouldn't it be great to blame our cravings on bacteria? And there are good reasons to do it. Our gut bacteria do communicate or "talk" to our brain and influence key neural centers that control our desire to eat. What we eat helps determine which species of bacteria thrive in our gut, so they have a strong motivation to influence our food choices.

Until recently, it has been thought that our appetite is solely controlled by centers in the brain. We know that there are specific hormones that trigger these centers and two are particularly important. The hormone ghrelin (from the Indo-European root *ghre*, to grow) is produced in cells in the stomach when it is empty. It is called the "hunger hormone." The second hormone, leptin, (from the Greek word *leptos*, which means thin) is produced by fat cells when we are full. It is called the "satiety hormone."

Ghrelin is the "ON" switch for eating, while leptin is the "OFF" switch to stop eating. Ghrelin stimulates the appetite; leptin decreases it.

The evolutionary values of these hormones are clear. If we have ample stores of nutrients, leptin turns down our drive to eat. If we run out of food, then ghrelin kicks in and we begin to hunt and gather. Our modern world confuses these hormones. If we stay up late, for example, and don't get enough sleep, it causes leptin to decrease so that we tend to eat more than we need and eventually gain weight.

There are other hormones and chemicals that also influence our appetite, including gastrin, secretin, cholecystokinin, gastric inhibitory peptide, and motilin. It turns out that gut bacteria produce hormones and chemicals that are very similar to leptin, ghrelin, and the others. We don't know for certain if the gut bacteria use these hormones to communicate with our brain and control our appetite, but indirect evidence from animal studies suggests that they do.

For example, researchers have injected mice with proteins produced by the bacteria *E. coli*, which is naturally found in the gut, and remarkably, the mice reduced their intake of food. It didn't matter whether they had previously eaten or they were hungry. In both cases, they refused food. The researchers found that the *E. coli* caused the release of a gut hormone associated with satiety, which stopped the mice from eating.

If human research determines that gut bacteria are the culprits responsible for our food obsessions, we would be one step closer to stopping the worldwide obesity epidemic. It would be much easier to restore the balance of our gut bacteria and naturally control our appetite and cravings than to go on a crash diet or rely on our sometimes nonexistent willpower to stop ourselves from devouring the next chocolate bar.

Gut Rap Q & A:

H Bomb: I hate the idea of a bacteria controlling me and influencing what I eat!

Doc Gut: Bacteria have had several billion years to figure out how to exploit their environment, and our gut is one of their favorite environments.

Ms. Natural: Are my gut bacteria responsible for my addictions?

Doc Gut: Right now we have to take responsibility. We know there are centers in the brain and specific neurotransmitters, like dopamine, involved with addictions, but we don't know how the gut bacteria might influence these neurotransmitters.

Ms. Natural: If fecal transplant can affect obesity, can it also affect appetite?

Doc Gut: Good question; I wish we knew the answer. We know that fecal transplant can affect obesity in animals by changing the types of bacteria present in the gut. And it is hypothesized that bacteria can influence our feelings of hunger and how much fat our body stores. So the answer to your question is that, in principle, they're related, but the details of how fecal transplant can change appetite in humans is still unknown.

Ms. Natural: Can you tell us more about ghrelin?

Doc Gut: Ghrelin is a hormone with many functions. It can increase the production of growth hormone (GH), lower the resistance of the blood vessels, and increase the output of the heart. It also stimulates the secretion of stomach acid and the movement of food.

Ghrelin levels increase when a person is fasting, which fits its role as a hunger hormone. It's also lower in individuals with a higher body weight compared to lean individuals. Researchers have been trying to figure out if it's involved in the regulation of body weight. But there's an odd contradiction. Ghrelin levels are higher in people who are thin and lower in obese people.

Ms. Natural: Is ghrelin affected by the kind of food we eat?

Doc Gut: Yes. Carbohydrates and proteins, for example, decrease the production and release of ghrelin more than fats.

Ms. Natural: What happens if we are dieting?

Doc Gut: Dieting has a similar effect to fasting. Since there is less food in the stomach, ghrelin increases and we get hungry, which makes it hard for us to stay on a diet.

H Bomb: What if I do something drastic like gastric bypass surgery?

Doc Gut: People who have had that surgery have been shown to have lower levels of ghrelin, which might explain why it's so successful.

H Bomb: I read somewhere that the bacteria that cause ulcers can affect ghrelin.

Doc Gut: The bacteria you are talking about is *Helicobacter pylori* or *H. pylori*, which was discovered to be one of the prime causes of peptic ulcers in the stomach. As a result of this finding, many people have been cured of ulcers in a matter of weeks with a simple treatment of antibiotics.

Researchers have found that *H. pylori* can also affect the levels of ghrelin in the blood. One study discovered that the levels of ghrelin and leptin increased after the *H. pylori* were eradicated and there was also an increase in body mass index (BMI). Does this mean destroying *H. pylori* in the stomach might create an increased risk of obesity? Only future research can answer this question.

REFERENCES:

Fetissov, SO, Role of the gut microbiota in host appetite control: bacterial growth to animal feeding behavior. *Nature Reviews Endocrinology* 2017; 13,11–25

Queipo-Ortuno, MI et al., Gut Microbiota Composition in Male Rat Models under Different Nutritional Status and Physical Activity and Its Association with Serum Leptin and Ghrelin Levels. *PLoS ONE* 2013; 8(5): e65465

Corfe, BM et al., The multifactorial interplay of diet, the microbiome and appetite control: current knowledge and future challenges. *Proceeding of the Nutrition Society* 2015; 74, (3). 235-244

Alcock, J et al., Is eating behavior manipulated by the gastrointestinal microbiota? Evolutionary pressures and potential mechanisms. *Bioessays* 2014; 36: 940–949

Norris, V et al., Hypothesis: Bacteria Control Host Appetites.*Journal of Bacteriology* February 2013; 195, 3, 411–416

Yakabi, K et al., Ghrelin and gastric acid secretion. *World Journal of Gastroenterology* 2008; 14(41):6334-6338

Khosravi, Y et al., Helicobacter pylori and gut microbiota modulate energy homeostasis prior to inducing histopathological changes in mice. *Gut Microbes* 2016; 7(1):48-53

CHAPTER 19

Epigenetics

Epigenetics is one of the most exciting new fields in modern medicine. When I told this to a friend, he informed me that the word "epigenetics" sounds intimidatingly scientific. I explained that epigenetics is simply the study of how genes are turned on and off and he changed his mind.

Every single thing we do turns our genes on and off—taking the dog for a walk, eating pizza, watching TV. Even prayer and meditation activate our genes.

To understand epigenetics more fully it helps to define a few terms. Each cell in our body contains DNA (except red blood cells). DNA, or deoxyribonucleic acid, is a molecule that carries the hereditary material and genetic instruction used in the growth, development, functioning, and reproduction of all known living organisms. There are 3 billion bits of information encoded in our human DNA.

The DNA consists of about 22,000 genes, which act as highly condensed micro-pieces of information that ultimately regulate all the different parts of the body.

The DNA is too small to see with a microscope. What we can see are larger structures called chromosomes. We have 23 pairs of chromosomes, each consisting of a single long strand of tightly wound DNA, surrounded by special proteins. The largest chromosome is called chromosome 1, and contains about 8,000 genes. The smallest is chromosome 21, containing fewer than 300 genes.

How do genes work? Not all of the 22,000 genes in each cell are active. As we said, some genes are turned on and others are turned off. A liver cell has genes that are turned on in order to detoxify toxins, while a white blood cell has genes turned on to protect us from invading microorganisms.

What is it that controls which genes are turned on or off in each cell? The answer to this question leads us to the famous debate: Nature versus Nurture.

Some scientists believed that our development from a single egg to an aged adult is controlled by a preprogrammed set of instructions in our DNA—Nature. Others argue that it is our environment that determines our development—Nurture. We now understand that both viewpoints are correct. Our genes are preprogrammed, but their expression can be modified by changes in the environment.

The process of turning genes on and off is called gene expression, and the study of gene expression is called epigenetics. One type of epigenetic phenomenon, for example, is how different foods turn our genes on and off. Some food helps prevent cardiovascular disease by altering gene expression. Studies have discovered how the omega-6 essential fatty acids turn on genes that cause inflammation, and how omega-3 essential fatty acids turn on genes that stop inflammation. Researchers are trying to alter the ratio of omega-3 to omega-6 essential fatty acids with diet and supplements to determine if this change can stop chronic inflammation and reduce or prevent heart attacks. So far, some studies say yes, while others are not so clear.

What does all this science have to do with gut bacteria? Gut bacteria use epigenetics. They produce chemicals that can turn genes on and off. For example, gut bacteria make folate, butyrate, biotin, and acetate, which enter the bloodstream and influence gene expression in many different cells. This is extremely important because if gut bacteria can influence our genes and DNA, they can influence everything that goes on in our bodies.

Modern research has demonstrated that our diet affects our gut bacteria, which in turn affects epigenetics and our health. Science is now discovering the underlying epigenetic mechanisms of the ancient dictum, "Food is medicine."

Gut Rap Q & A:

H Bomb: Doc, did you really say that food can help prevent cancer?

Doc Gut: Yes. Nutrigenomics is a science that studies how food affects our genes. Food components, such as polyphenols, isothiocyanates, folate, selenium, retinoids, and fatty acids help prevent the development of cancer by influencing gene expression. Cruciferous vegetables like broccoli and Brussels sprouts, for example, contain isothiocyanates, which have been shown to detoxify many types of carcinogens.

Ms. Natural: What about herbal supplements?

Dr. Doctor: The field of nutrigenomics extends to the study of herbal supplements. The herb echinacea, for example, has been shown to turn certain genes on and off. It can turn on interferon producing genes that help protect the body from bad microorganisms. It can also turn off inflammation-related genes. Other spices also do this. Turmeric and ginger can beneficially affect a wide number of important genes, including turning off genes that may cause chronic inflammation or cancer.

Ms. Natural: Does epigenetics explain why one person gets sick and another doesn't?

Doc Gut: In many ways, it does. One interesting study in the field of epigenetics looked at gene expression in response to a viral infection. A group of healthy adults was inoculated with Influenza A virus. Blood samples were taken for several days before and after the inoculation and results showed that some people in the group got sick while others didn't. Those who did not get sick had a different pattern of gene expression. In other words, they had a different set of genes turned on than the people who got sick.

Ms. Natural: What exactly is the genetic code?

Doc Gut: The genetic code is a set of rules that allows a particular sequence of biochemicals in the DNA to be translated into a specific sequence of amino acids in a protein. These proteins are either used to form structures in the body or to create enzymes. Enzymes are crucial. They direct all the biochemical pathways in our cells. The DNA ultimately uses enzymes to tell every part of our body what to do.

Ms. Natural: Do we all have the same genes?

Doc Gut: Except for identical twins, every person is unique. We inherit half of our genes from our mother and half from our father. The complete set of genes of each individual is called a genome.

Ms. Natural: We hear a lot about the "Human Genome Project." What is it?

Doc Gut: The word genome is defined as the total collection of genes in any individual. The Human Genome Project was a scientific investigation that eventually identified and decoded all of the genes in human DNA, including vast regions (98%) within the DNA called non-coding DNA. These regions used to be called "junk DNA," but we now realize that they are critical and contain instructions on when and how certain genes need to be turned on and off in each cell.

Ms. Natural: Are our genes different from the ones our gut bacteria have?

Doc Gut: Yes and no. We have, as we said, about 22,000 genes encoded in our DNA. The gut bacteria collectively have about 8,000,000 genes, about 360 times more. So they obviously have many more different types of genes than we do. However, researchers have found certain bacterial DNA sequences in the human genome.

Ms. Natural: How did they get there?

Doc Gut: No one knows.

Ms. Natural: You mentioned that meditation can create epigenetic effects.

Doc Gut: Yes. The research I'm most familiar with shows that the Transcendental Meditation® (TM®) program affects the expression of over 70 genes. Another exciting study, which was partially funded by the National Institutes of Health, reveals that regular practice of the TM program increases expression of a specific gene that could even help reverse the aging process.

REFERENCES:

Zaina, S and Lund, G, Epigenetics: A Tool to Understand Diet-Related Cardiovascular Risk. *J. Nutrigenet Nutrigenomics* 2011; 4:261–274

Ong, TP et al., Targeting the Epigenome with Bioactive Food Components for Cancer Prevention. *J Nutrigenet Nutrigenomics* 2011; 4:275–292

Randolph, RK et al., Regulation of Human Immune Gene Expression as Influenced by a Commercial Blended Echinacea Product: Preliminary Studies. *Experimental Biology and Medicine* 2003; 228:1051-1056

Tiwari, AK et al., Pharmacogenetics of anxiolytic drugs. *J Neural Transm* 2009; 116:667–677

Huang, Y et al., Temporal Dynamics of Host Molecular Responses Differentiate Symptomatic and Asymptomatic Influenza A Infection. *PLoS Genet* 2011; 7(8): e1002234

Duraimani, S et al., Effects of Lifestyle Modification on Telomerase Gene Expression in Hypertensive Patients: A Pilot Trial of Stress Reduction and Health Education Programs in African Americans. *PLoS ONE* 2015; 10(11): e0142689

Wenuganen, S, Anti-Aging Effects of the Transcendental Meditation Program: Analysis of Ojas Level and Global Gene Expression. Maharishi University of Management, ProQuest Dissertations Publishing, 3630467, 2014

Maharishi Ayurveda and Vedic Technology: Creating Ideal Health for the Individual and World, Adapted and Updated from The Physiology of Consciousness: Part 2 by Robert Keith Wallace, PhD, Dharma Publications, 2016

Prasher, B et al., Whole genome expression and biochemical correlates of extreme constitutional types defined in Ayurveda. *Journal of Translational Medicine* 2008; 6:48

Lantza, RC et al., The effect of extracts from ginger rhizome on inflammatory mediator production. *Phytomedicine* 2007; 14 123–128

Hullar, MAJ and Fu, BC, Diet, the Gut Microbiome, and Epigenetics. Cancer journal (Sudbury, Mass). 2014; 20(3):170-175

Riley, DR et al., Bacteria-human somatic cell lateral gene transfer is enriched in cancer samples. *PLOS Computational Biology* June 2013

CHAPTER 20

Prebiotics

We know about antibiotics, we know about probiotics, but what the heck are prebiotics? A prebiotic is a fibrous food that promotes the growth of friendly gut bacteria. The prebiotic resists both stomach acid and the digestive enzymes in our small intestine, and therefore passes into our large intestine where it is digested and fermented by beneficial gut bacteria.

We spoke briefly about different prebiotic foods before and some may already be common in our diet, for instance, asparagus, wheat bran, bananas, garlic, onions, and leeks. We may be slightly less familiar with prebiotics like Jerusalem artichokes, dandelion greens, and chicory root. One of the main ingredients in all of them is a substance called inulin (used commercially to add bulk to many processed foods).

Research has shown that prebiotics, as well as probiotics, can help patients with ulcerative colitis. They appear to help in the absorption of calcium and other minerals, and both animal and human studies suggest that prebiotics improve immune function. There is also evidence that prebiotics may help people with high blood pressure or type 2 diabetes, as well as decreasing childhood infection. A promising new area of research focuses on the potential benefits of prebiotics for colorectal cancer.

Some studies have examined the psychological and neurological effects of prebiotics. Mice given prebiotics showed enhanced associative learning and working memory. Prebiotics can also increase an important chemical in the nervous system called brain-derived neurotropic factor, or BDNF, which helps nerve cells to grow and mature.

You might wonder how prebiotics are able to produce all these benefits, but the exact mechanisms are not yet known. It's suggested that the prebiotics feed specific friendly bacteria in our lower gut and make them stronger. These good bacteria then produce chemical messengers, which enter our bloodstream and use epigenetic mechanisms (see previous chapter) to switch on genes that alter chemical pathways to create a variety of positive effects.

Not all prebiotics are good for everyone. As we learned in a previous chapter, fibrous foods can cause gas in some people, especially if their gut is damaged.

Gut Rap Q & A:

H Bomb: What's up with bloating?

Doc Gut: Bloating is very common in certain digestive disorders and is due to a build up of gas in the GI tract, which is not immediately released. Some bacteria are strong gas producers; others are not. Some food ferments quickly, and some slowly. So if you do have bloating it could be due to a number of factors.

Ms. Natural: Why are prebiotics considered to be good if they cause the growth of bacteria in the lower gut that could result in the production of excess gas and bloating?

Doc Gut: The prebiotics help some people because the bacteria in their gut can slowly ferment and digest these substances to produce beneficial substances such as short-chained fatty acids. Other people may have some form of IBS, and, as a result, they are more sensitive to the build up of excess gas. They should probably avoid prebiotic gas-producing foods.

H Bomb: I once worked with a guy who farted probably twenty times a day, and they were whoppers. Should we blame them on his lower gut bacteria or the prebiotics he might be eating?

Doc Gut: Both. It's not abnormal to fart or, to be more polite, pass wind. This is just a natural way of releasing the excess gas produced by our gut bacteria during the process of fermentation. Healthy women pass wind about seven times a day, and men do it twice as much. It can be uncomfortable to hold in excess gas.

It extends your abdomen and causes further pain. The amount of gas released either by farting or belching depends on many factors, including the state of your gut bacteria, the intake of prebiotic foods, and whether your gut walls are intact or leaky.

REFERENCES:

Slavin, J, Fiber and Prebiotics: Mechanisms and Health Benefits. *Nutrients.* 2013; 5(4):1417-1435

Yoo, JY and Kim, SS, Probiotics and Prebiotics: Present Status and Future Perspectives on Metabolic Disorders. *Nutrients* 2016; 8(3):173

Di Bartolometo, F, Prebiotics to fight diseases: reality or fiction. *Phytother Res* 2013; 10, 1457-1473

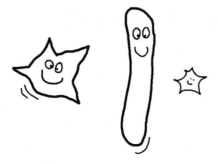

PART 4

DOC GUT'S FAVORITE BOOKS

CHAPTER 21

The Brain Maker

Dr. David Perlmutter is one of the most popular doctors in the field of alternative medicine. He is a qualified neurologist as well as a pioneer in the use of diet and probiotics to improve health. He believes in evidence-based medicine and includes the most advanced integrative research findings.

In his earlier book *Grain Brain*, he warns about the perils of modern wheat for many neurological disorders, and he recommends a completely gluten-free diet. He also explains why cholesterol is critical for our brain and cites many studies that disagree with the long-held belief that fat and cholesterol are bad for our health.

In *The Brain Maker*, Dr. Perlmutter focuses on the microbiome and how it affects our health. He includes many personal accounts of patients suffering from severe neurological disorders who were helped by his treatment programs, which include a gluten-free diet, probiotics, and changes in lifestyle.

Dr. Perlmutter tells us how foods containing gluten disrupt the gut bacteria and trigger a leaky gut. Normally, the gut wall is able to prevent substances from leaving the gut and entering our bloodstream, but a poor diet and a disrupted state of gut bacteria (which can be due to excess sugar) cause the junctions between the cells in the lining to open, creating "leaks" in the gut wall.

Lipopolysaccharide or LPS is a natural component of the outer membrane of a certain class of bacteria (Gram-negative bacteria) that are sometimes present in the gut. When these bacteria are destroyed and their cell walls break apart, they release LPS into the gut. If a person has a leaky gut, it has been suggested by alternative doctors that the LPS enters the bloodstream, causing a severe immune response and inflammation throughout the body. The release of LPS into the bloodstream in a severe bacterial infection is well documented, and results in septic shock. It is estimated that there are more than 1,000,000 cases of sepsis among hospitalized patients each year in the US.

Dr. Perlmutter cites several studies in which LPS was injected into animals, resulting in both learning deficits and memory problems. In human studies, Alzheimer's patients were found to have three times as much LPS in their blood as healthy controls. Patients with ALS (also known as Lou Gehrig's disease) have higher levels of LPS, and these levels correlate with the severity of the disease. New findings also reveal unusually high levels of LPS in patients with Parkinson's disease.

Another interesting topic is the effect of glyphosate, the active ingredient in the herbicide Roundup, on gut bacteria. Dr. Perlmutter explains that it is estimated that by 2017, farmers will have applied a remarkable 1.35 million metric tons of glyphosate to their crops. He suggests that glyphosate is affecting gluten sensitivity, and that the rise in gluten intolerance and celiac disease may be due to the increased use of this chemical.

He also refers to research on the effects of glyphosate in the body by MIT scientist Dr. Stephanie Seneff and a coworker. In a report published in the *Journal of Interdisciplinary Toxicology,* they point out that glyphosate can inhibit an enzyme produced by gut bacteria that helps detoxify many chemicals. The result could be that the intestinal wall is compromised and harmful substances are able to get into the bloodstream. In addition, the authors explain how glyphosate can disrupt a critical pathway (the shikimate pathway) in bacteria for making neurotransmitters and important biochemicals, as well as altering the balance between pathogens and beneficial bacteria in the gut. The scientists imply that glyphosate might be the single most important cause of the rise in gluten sensitivity.

Dr. Perlmutter's advice is to radically change our diet, eat organic foods and grass-fed animals, and take probiotics, orally or in an enema, to help heal our gut lining. The probiotic enema is one of his most successful treatment tools, helping patients with otherwise incurable neurological disorders.

His website (www.drperlmutter.com) has some fascinating interviews with several of the main movers and shakers in the alternative health world.

Gut Rap Q & A:

Ms. Natural: What does Dr. Perlmutter say about sugar and neurological disorders?

Doc Gut: In both his books, he explains how sugar can cause inflammation, which is the basis of many different neurological disorders. Excess sugar triggers a reaction called glycation, during which the sugar becomes attached to proteins and fats, creating what he calls "deformed molecules." (The technical term for these molecules is "advanced glycation end products" or AGEs.) Dr. Perlmutter says that the correlation between poor sugar control and Alzheimer's disease is so prominent that it's referred to as "type-3 diabetes."

Ms. Natural: Would you tell us how to do a probiotic enema?

Doc Gut: In his book, *The Brain Maker,* Dr. Perlmutter lists what you need for a probiotic enema: an enema bag or enema bulb, as well as a good probiotic supplement that preferably includes a large number of *Bifidobacteria.* You start by making sure you have a complete bowel elimination. The next step is to make the probiotic mixture. Dr. Perlmutter suggests using 3 to 6 probiotic capsules or 1/8 teaspoon powdered probiotic, and mixing this with 12 ounces of lukewarm water. The easiest and safest place to take the enema is in your bathtub. Dr. Perlmutter recommends holding the enema in for 30 minutes, if possible (emphasis on IF).

For severe problems, he has prescribed as many as three enemas a week for 4 to 6 weeks.

H Bomb: What does Dr. Perlmutter say about the substances the gut bacteria produce?

Doc Gut: He explains that gut bacteria make brain-derived neurotrophic factor (BDNF), which is important to the brain because it helps in the creation of new cells in the brain and it also protects existing brain cells. Lower levels are found in a number of neurological disorders, including Alzheimer's disease.

He also discusses the different short-chain fatty acids (SCFAs) that bacteria produce. The three main ones are acetic, propionic, and butyric. Butyric is an important energy source for the cells lining the colon, and it is also anti-inflammatory and anti-carcinogenic. Different bacteria produce different SCFAs. The amount of each of these substances depends on the composition of the bacteria and the diet.

One of these SCFAs, he explains, can even be toxic to the brain. This is propionic acid or PPA, which is produced by certain types of *Clostridia* bacteria. Why is PPA bad? PPA can increase intestinal permeability, creating a leaky gut problem. PPA can then get into the bloodstream and cause an inflammatory response, disrupt the way cells communicate with each other, and damage cell parts including membranes and DNA. In one study, PPA has even been shown to trigger symptoms of autism. The good news, however, is that researchers have found substances that can counter the effects of PPA.

Ms. Natural: What do you think of the documentary
What's with Wheat?

Doc Gut: It's a comprehensive and easy to understand presentation that explains why wheat is the cause of celiac disease and gluten sensitivity. Dr. Perlmutter is featured in the documentary, along with several other prominent doctors, scientists, and health experts. They are all very sincere and provide strong arguments why wheat and gluten are the main cause of many of today's diseases. This is a controversial issue but the scientific evidence presented is compelling. The description of how wheat has been hybridized and treated extensively with glyphosate and other chemicals is especially interesting.

REFERENCES:

The Brain Maker: The Power of Gut Microbes to Heal and Protect Your Brain by Dr. David Perlmutter, Little, Brown and Company, 2015

Grain Brain: The Surprising Truth about Wheat, Carbs, and Sugar— Your Brain's Silent Killers by David Perlmutter and Kristin Loberg, Little, Brown and Company, 2013

Lee, YJ et al., Inhibitory effect of 4-O-methylhonokiol on lipopolysaccharide-induced neuroinflammation amyloidogenesis and memory impairment via inhibition of nuclear factor-kappaB in vitro and in vivo models. *J Neuroinflammation* 2012; 9:35

Canny, GO, and McCormick, BA, Bacteria in the Intestine, Helpful Residents or Enemies from Within? *Infect. Immun* 2008; 76, (8), 3360-3373

Martin, GS, Sepsis, severe sepsis and septic shock: changes in incidence, pathogens and outcomes. *Expert review of anti-infective therapy* 2012; 10(6):701-706

Samsel, A and Seneff, S, Glyphosate, pathways to modern diseases II: Celiac sprue and gluten intolerance. *Interdiscip Toxicol* 2013: 6(4): 159–184

Samsel, A and Seneff, S, Glyphosate's suppression of cytochrome P450 enzymes and amino acid biosynthesis by the gut microbiome: Pathways to modern diseases. *Entropy* 2013: 15: 1416–1463

The documentary *What's with Wheat?* is currently available on Netflix.

CHAPTER 22

The Microbiome Solution

In *The Microbiome Solution* Dr. Robynne Chutkan gives a comprehensive overview of specific factors that disrupt our gut bacteria. She explains that while antibiotics have saved millions of lives, the medical profession now recognizes that they have been over-used. She explains that in the US and other developed countries, a combination of excessive antibiotics combined with ultra hygienic indoor environments has left us vulnerable to auto-immune and chronic health conditions, which can all be traced back to an imbalance in gut bacteria.

Dr. Chutkan offers practical programs to restore the balance of our gut bacteria and improve our health. Her recommendations range from diet and lifestyle changes to specific probiotics and supplements. She talks about how to choose a probiotic and explains that since bacteria naturally compete with each other, it's important for us to have the right combination. She describes choosing a probiotic that has seven different compatible strains that include *Lactobacilli* and *Bifidobacteria*. She also suggests that we use one that has at least 50 billion CFU or colony-forming units.

She explains that we should look carefully at the shelf life or expiration date, and whether or not the probiotic needs to be refrigerated. Dr. Chutkan advises that we use only manufacturers who guarantee that their products have been properly tested and contain the amount of live bacteria stated on the label.

Probiotics are a highly unregulated area, so it's best to check the Internet to see if any clinical trials have been done using the bacteria listed on the label. She also explains that some people may not see results for some time if they have too much damage in their gut.

Dr. Chutkan also talks about fecal transplants and the latest findings on their success under different conditions. One of her personal favorite recommendations is to raise your children on a farm, where they can naturally be exposed to different kinds of bacteria. At the end of *The Microbiome Solution* she provides appealing and practical recipes that incorporate her many suggestions.

Gut Rap Q & A:

H Bomb: Is this Dr. Chutkan another health quack?

Doc Gut: No, she is a well-trained gastroenterologist, and her advice is supported by strong research and clinical experience.

Ms. Natural: Does she say how long it takes before we can experience results implementing her treatment programs?

Doc Gut: Dr. Chutkan is very honest and tells us that the improvement of our symptoms depends on many factors, especially the extent of damage in our gut.

Ms. Natural: Does she recommend any specific probiotic?

Doc Gut: Dr. Chutkan specifically recommends a formulation called VSL#3, which has been shown to reduce inflammatory bowel disease, and says that some of her own patients who took this noticed improvements. She tells us that the longer we've been taking antibiotics, the longer it will take to restore our gut bacteria. She also agrees with many doctors who feel that we may have to continue probiotics indefinitely to maintain gut health.

H Bomb: What's the point of probiotics? The stomach or intestinal enzymes may destroy them even before they reach the lower gut.

Doc Gut: That's true. She does say that some probiotics just pass through the gut and are excreted, so they aren't very effective. But some companies take this into account and cover their probiotics with a special enteric coating, which allows them to survive the stomach acids. If you experience any sort of benefit, you can assume that at least some of the good guys reached your gut and are working to make you healthier.

H Bomb: Okay, let's say by some slim chance that they make it to the lower gut, how do they survive the raging warfare with all the other billions of bacteria fighting for dominance? It seems like sending elementary school kids to play in the Super Bowl.

Doc Gut: There are studies that show distinct benefits from taking probiotics for patients with digestive disorders. We will just have to wait until all the clinical trials are finished before we know how effective the different probiotics are for other conditions.

REFERENCES:

The Microbiome Solution: A Radical New Way to Heal Your body From Inside Out by Robynne Chutkan, MD, Penguin Random House, 2015

Ventola, CL, The Antibiotic Resistance Crisis: Part 1: Causes and Threats. *Pharmacy and Therapeutics* 2015; 40(4):277-283

Ventola CL, The Antibiotic Resistance Crisis: Part 2: Management Strategies and New Agents. *Pharmacy and Therapeutics* 2015; 40(5):344-352

CHAPTER 23

The Plant Paradox

The Plant Paradox by Dr. Steven Gundry offers new and interesting insights into gut repair. Dr. Gundry has unusual credentials for an expert in diet and digestion. He is the former Head of the Division of Cardiothoracic Surgery at Loma Linda University School of Medicine, performed pioneering pediatric heart transplants, invented new medical devices, and has published over 300 articles and book chapters on his research. He is also the author of *Dr. Gundry's Diet Evolution*.

The Plant Paradox explains that lectins are the most evil offenders in our digestive health woes. Lectins are usually defined as special proteins that tend to bind with carbohydrates on the surface of different cells. They are found in many plant products, as well as in our own body. Dr. Gundry identifies two particularly harmful lectins in wheat, which are gluten and wheat germ agglutinin or WGA. Gluten is usually considered a storage protein. WGA is a well-known lectin and research has shown that it can cause digestive problems. Other foods such as tomatoes, beans, cashews, and peanuts are also high in lectins.

So we can't have gluten-free pasta or tomatoes. Cancel our trip to Italy!

What on earth *can* we eat? His books answer this and other questions and he offers a wide selection of recipes, tips, and interesting bits of new knowledge. For example, eating a handful of raw red kidney beans can kill us. This is because of the large amount of lectins in them. However, if we cook them thoroughly in a pressure cooker, it breaks down the lectins and makes kidney beans safe to eat.

Dr. Gundry, like other experts before him, maintains that disease begins in the gut. His diet and supplement program is designed to stop the gut from being damaged and to heal it. As he explains, many grasses and plants naturally produce lectins to protect themselves from insects and animals. Some grazing animals have evolved physiological mechanisms to deal with the bad effects lectins produce in the stomach. Unfortunately, we have not.

Lectins, Dr. Gundry tells us, act like thorns in our gut. They damage the gut lining and cause leaky gut syndrome. Ultimately, this leads to an overactive immune system and autoimmune diseases like rheumatoid arthritis. Everyone is lectin sensitive to a degree, and some of us to a much greater extent.

Dr. Gundry has a lot more to say about which foods are good for us and which are bad. He describes "killer genes" that are turned on by calorie-rich food, and which lead to the major killers, including heart disease and cancer. He compares the ecology of our gut bacteria to a rainforest and explains that if we napalm this rainforest with antibiotics, it takes many years to grow back and fully restore

166

itself. In the meantime, the bad bacteria take over the rainforest and tell our brain what they want to eat.

The good guys are still present, but they are hiding and in much smaller numbers. Unless we change our diet, Dr. Gundry tells us, they have no chance to regain their natural healthy dominance. Probiotics are a very temporary solution, lasting only two weeks according to Dr. Gundry. He explains that we must feed the good guys prebiotics. And not just any prebiotic. He has created his own formula with special prebiotics to feed the good guys, and other ingredients to knock out the bad bugs. According to Dr. Gundry, the bad guys love sugar, so as long as they are in power, they are constantly sending messages to the brain to eat more and more sugar. The result is that not only do we gain weight, but the bad bugs in our gut reign supreme.

Gut Rap Q & A

Ms. Natural: How do we know that this isn't just part of another new fad?

Doc Gut: Excellent question. The situation is confusing. I'm not sure why doctors got it so wrong in the past. They told us not to eat too much butter or eggs because those would elevate our cholesterol, and to use margarine instead. But now that research is being challenged and sugar and gluten are the new bad guys. Was it because of poor research? Yes. Did the food industries pressure them to favor one type of food and not another? They did. How do we find our way through these often confusing information minefields?

Dr. Gundry and others are challenging very strongly held beliefs. Civilization was built on the ability to grow and store grains in order to have food for the winter months. We could almost say that being addicted to bread, pasta, cookies, and cakes is part of our cultural heritage.

If Dr. Gundry is correct, it will have a huge effect on the food industry. There is still very little research that has been done on the effect of lectins on humans. Dr. Gundry did some research a few years ago, but it is not yet well known, and as far as I can tell it was only presented at conferences and has not yet been published in a peer-review journal. And I have not seen any published research on his special prebiotic formula, although there is some research on the different components of it.

Dr. Gundry is not the only physician coming out with new gut recommendations, diets, and products. The Internet is full of information overload, and there is no way to determine which diets or supplements will benefit our health.

H Bomb: Are we humans so stupid that we can't tell what we should and shouldn't eat?

Doc Gut: Dr. Gundry says yes. He feels that our consumption of lectins over so many years has caused a plague on the health of mankind.

H Bomb: Isn't ricin a lectin? I know that in the late '70s, a Bulgarian political writer was assassinated in London when his leg was pierced with a micro-engineered pellet of ricin on the tip of an umbrella.

Doc Gut: You're right. Ricin is a lectin produced by the castor oil bean, and it's extremely deadly if injected or breathed in as a powder. The equivalent of only a few grains of salt is deadly. We don't have to worry about taking castor oil because heating during the process of oil extraction denatures and deactivates the ricin protein making it harmless and beneficial for several medicinal purposes.

H Bomb: Dr. Gundry calls gluten a lectin, but I have looked through a number of scientific papers and seen gluten and lectin referred to as two separate types of proteins.

Doc Gut: Identifying gluten as a lectin is rather unusual, although both gluten and lectins are considered "sticky proteins." Lectins are sticky because they bind to carbohydrates on certain receptors located on the cell membrane. Gluten is sticky because it contains two proteins (prolamin and glutelin) that bind together to form an elastic-like substance that traps gas and gives bread its chewy texture and body. Gluten could be considered to have lectin-like qualities since it binds to receptors on gut cells.

**Ms. Natural: Does Dr. Gundry say anything about
H. pylori bacteria?**

Doc Gut: He says there are two types of *H. pylori.* One is a pathological type that can cause ulcers in certain people, and the other is a nonpathological type, which has beneficial effects. The nonpathological type, Dr. Gundry explains, may actually be helpful in losing weight. It does this by normalizing acid secretion and reducing the production of the hormone ghrelin in the stomach. Ghrelin, as we mentioned, signals the brain to eat more.

**H Bomb: I've read Internet articles about these guys with their
leaky gut theories. Some people call them quacks because they
use animal studies to make a case for their diet recommendations
and pricey products. They also tend to use testimonials from
individuals and celebrities, and have special promotional sales.
They just sound untrustworthy to me.**

Doc Gut: The salesmanship may be excessive but they are not quacks. They often have very good credentials and help many people. There's no doubt that Dr. Gundry is an excellent MD who has performed remarkable heart operations. He also has many interesting new ideas about diet and gut bacteria, some of which challenge current medical opinion.

REFERENCES:

YouTube videos: *Enter Dr. Steven Gundry's World of Gut Microbes,* https://www.youtube.com/watch?v=oOSJJSS4cnk

Dr. Gundry's Diet Evolution: Turn Off The Genes That Are Killing You And Your Waistline by Steven R. Gundry, M.D., Harmony, 2008

The Plant Paradox: The Hidden Dangers in "Healthy" Foods That Cause Disease and Weight Gain by Steven R. Gundry, M.D., Harper Wave, 2017

CHAPTER 24

Gut and Psychology Syndrome

One of the most influential books on the link between neurological, psychological, and digestive problems is *Gut and Psychology Syndrome* by Dr. Natasha Campbell-McBride, which we mentioned in the chapter *Brain Wiring*. She describes effective and lasting treatments for hundreds of children and adults with autistic spectrum disorders, attention deficit hyperactivity disorder (ADHD/ADD), schizophrenia, dyslexia, dyspraxia, depression, obsessive-compulsive disorder, bipolar disorder and other psychiatric problems.

Dr. Campbell-McBride recommends what is called the GAPS diet, which is named after the title of her book *Gut and Psychology Syndrome*. This program was derived from a diet created in the first half of the 20th century by Dr. Sidney Valentine Haas and his team for patients with celiac disease and other digestive disorders. This original diet was called the Specific Carbohydrate Diet (SCD). Dr. Haas found that patients could tolerate proteins and fats but had difficulty with complex carbohydrates derived from grains, starchy vegetables, and sugars, especially lactose or milk sugar. In

1951, Dr. Haas's diet was published in the medical textbook *The Management of Celiac Disease*, and was highly regarded in the treatment of celiac patients.

Dr. Campbell-McBride explains that an interesting turn of events happened. In the 1950s, celiac disease was discovered to be a gluten intolerance condition, and its primary treatment program was a gluten-free diet. People with other digestive conditions, who had previously been included with celiac patients, were no longer advised to follow the SCD diet. In 1994, the SCD diet regained its popularity with the publication of Elaine Gottschall's book *Breaking the Vicious Cycle: Intestinal Health Through Diet*, which described her experiences using this diet to heal her child who had ulcerative colitis and neurological problems.

Gut and Psychology Syndrome includes a summary of the history of research connecting neurological conditions with digestive disorders and gut bacteria. The book offers a practical treatment plan, which starts with a simple bone broth to heal the gut lining. According to Dr. Campbell-McBride, bone broth is filled with nutrient-dense foods that feed the friendly gut bacteria and give the intestinal lining a chance to rest and heal. The subsequent stages of the plan gradually introduce different types of foods until the full GAPS diet is prescribed.

There are many health practitioners today who use either this diet or variations of it to heal the gut. Dr. Campbell-McBride, who holds a degree in Medicine, and postgraduate degrees in both Neurology and Human Nutrition, has started an entire move-ment based on the idea that there's a vital need to detoxify and rebalance the gut in order for our brains to develop and function properly. She points out that many of us, while not being celiac patients, do have a sensitivity to grains and milk. Her diet is recommended for anyone with digestive problems, as well as many other health conditions.

Dr. Campbell-McBride talks briefly about two important proteins that have to be broken down—gluten from wheat and casein from milk. If gluten and casein are not properly broken down, they can be converted into opiate-like substances called casomorphin and gliadomorphin, which are believed to disrupt the development and activity of the brain and adversely affect children with autism and schizophrenia.

A far more current discussion of the effects of diet on schizophrenia, autism, and other mental conditions can be found in an article entitled *Bread and Other Edible Agents of Mental Disease*, which was published in a respected scientific journal by two professors from the University of Padua, Italy. The opiate-like substances from the improper digestion of gluten and casein are referred to as exorphins. Exorphins bind to opioid receptors and affect the state of the brain. They can be both addictive and hallucinogenic. The exorphins are related to endorphins, which are our body's natural painkillers and are said to be responsible for a "runner's high."

When these exorphins are injected into mice, their behavior becomes restless, then inactive, and then hyper-defensive. Schizophrenic and autistic patients have been shown to have higher levels of these substances, and when given a grain and milk free diet, they improve. The authors point out that even though individual patients can show marked recovery on these diets, they are unwilling to continue them because the foods are so addicting.

Gut Rap Q & A:

Ms. Natural: Can you tell us more about Elaine Gottschall?

Doc Gut: On the official website of her book, *Breaking the Vicious Cycle*, there is a wonderful story about how she had to fight the doctors of her time who wanted to remove most of her young daughter's colon, forcing the child to forever wear an external bag for waste products. She sought out the elderly Dr. Haas and asked for his advice. He told her to change the child's diet. Ten days later, her daughter's neurological problems improved. After a few months her digestive problems also improved and in two years she was free of all symptoms. Mrs. Gottschall went on to receive degrees in the biological sciences, and at her husband's urging wrote her now famous book, which has had a huge impact on many people.

Ms. Natural: What does Dr. Campbell-McBride say about supplements?

Doc Gut: She feels that most supplements aren't absorbed very well into our system, especially if you have leaky gut syndrome. Also, nutrients can compete for absorption sites so if you take supplements you need to be careful how you combine them. For example, too much calcium might make it difficult for other minerals like magnesium, zinc, or iron to be absorbed.

Ms. Natural: What is the difference between synthetic and natural supplements?

Doc Gut: This is a controversial subject. Most doctors and scientists say that there is no difference, but alternative health experts disagree, based on their clinical experience. Unfortunately, there are no carefully controlled scientific studies to help clarify the issue.

Ms. Natural: Does Dr. Campbell-McBride have you stop taking supplements when you start her diet?

Doc Gut: No. But she recommends that you check the ingredients carefully to make sure that they don't conflict with her diet and harm your gut. If you want to take supplements, she prefers that you take them in liquid form because it has a higher absorption rate. She suggests supplements with fulvic acid, which also helps absorption. Her preference is to obtain vitamins and nutrients from natural sources. For example, Dr. Campbell-McBride highly recommends cod liver oil as a means to ingest omega-3-essential fatty acids, cholesterol, and vitamins A and D, pointing out that it has provided benefits for centuries, and is especially useful for children with gut problems.

H Bomb: What does she say about stomach acid?
I have way too much acid.

Doc Gut: She explains that stomach acid is important for the digestion of proteins. If the pH of our stomach isn't acidic enough, then the enzyme pepsin will not be activated and fail to do its job of both breaking down proteins into smaller units and triggering two important digestive hormones, secretin and cholecystokinin.

Secretin tells the stomach to stop producing acid and signals the liver to start producing bile to help in fat digestion. It also tells the pancreas to produce bicarbonate to neutralize stomach acids and make the pH of the small intestine more alkaline so that the pancreatic digestive enzymes can do their job.

Cholecystokinin also has several important functions. It tells the gallbladder to release the bile for fat digestion and tells the stomach to stop its activity. Finally and most importantly, it signals the pancreas to produce its digestive enzymes and to release them into the small intestine.

H Bomb: I guess that means she isn't into reducing stomach acid.

Doc Gut: No, she isn't. In fact, in certain cases, she actually recommends adding supplements to increase the stomach acid. She does this not only because it might help digestion but also to help balance gut bacteria. When the stomach doesn't have enough acid, she explains, certain opportunistic bacteria grow on the stomach wall and can play an important role in stomach cancer, as well as other conditions. Another problem is that if the pH is not low enough then these bacteria can digest the sugar in the stomach and produce gas, which can be very uncomfortable. She also feels that the bacteria can grow around the sphincter muscle and disturb its proper functions. As a result, the acid from the stomach goes up the esophagus, creating an acid reflux. Instead of trying to suppress stomach acid, she tries to enhance it.

Ms. Natural: What does Dr. Campbell-McBride think about taking digestive enzymes to help digestion?

Doc Gut: She feels that diet is far more important and does not recommend digestive enzymes. Based on her clinical experience, she emphasizes that diet is the best way to heal the gut.

H Bomb: You mentioned that she uses bone broth to heal the gut, but I read somewhere that bone broth was found to have a higher content of lead than plain water.

Doc Gut: Yes, one article suggests that bone broth made from organic chickens had a higher lead content than the water used to cook the chickens in. However, a very comprehensive group called the Weston A. Price Foundation has reviewed this article and shown that the lead levels were acceptable and were most likely a result of the study being done in an area of England that was contaminated with lead.

Ms. Natural: On a more mundane note, can you tell me the difference between broth and stock?

Doc Gut: Bone broth and stock are two different things. Bone broth is mostly bones, water, and some salt and pepper, perhaps with onions. Stock is meat and water. Stew includes vegetables and spices.

Ms. Natural: How does Dr. Campbell-McBride feel about being a vegetarian or vegan?

Doc Gut: She generally doesn't like it but says that a vegetarian diet, which includes animal foods such as dairy products and eggs, is fine. She is strongly against a purely plant based diet and feels that being a vegan is unhealthy and can only be justified as a type of short-term fasting or cleansing.

H Bomb: Do you agree with her?

Doc Gut: I agree with some things but not others. Being a vegetarian requires a certain amount of knowledge and is particularly challenging if you need to cut out grains. But I believe with a little information and care it is certainly possible to be a healthy vegetarian. It's much harder to be a vegan, but I understand why people who care about cows would choose this path.

REFERENCES:

Gut and Psychology Syndrome by Dr. Natasha Campbell-McBride, MD, Medinform Publishing Cambridge, UK, 2010, http://www.gapsdiet.com

Official website of Elaine Gottschall's book *Breaking the Vicious Cycle: Intestinal Health Through Diet* is http://www.breakingtheviciouscycle.info/home

Bressan, P and Kramer, P. Bread and Other Edible Agents of Mental Disease. *Frontiers in Human Neuroscience.* 2016; 10:130

See Wikipedia for more information on secretin and cholecystokinin.

See Wikipedia for more information on lactase.

Troelsen, JT et al., Regulation of lactase-phlorizin hydrolase gene expression by the caudal-related homoeodomain protein Cdx-2. *The Biochemical Journal* 1997; 322 (3) 833–8

Bersaglieri, T et al., Genetic signatures of strong recent positive selection at the lactase gene. *American Journal of Human Genetics* 2004; 74 (6):1111–20

Kuokkanen, M et al., Transcriptional regulation of the lactase-phlorizin hydrolase gene by polymorphisms associated with adult-type hypolactasia. *Gut* 2003; 52 (5): 647–52

Troelsen, JT, Adult-type hypolactasia and regulation of lactase expression. *Biochimica et Biophysica Acta* 2005; 1723 (1-3): 19–32

Wang, Y et al., The genetically programmed down-regulation of lactase in children. *Gastroenterology* 1998; 114 (6):1230–6

CHAPTER 25

The Prime

Dr. Kulreet Chaudhary is an Integrative neurologist, whose book, *The Prime,* offers an excellent introduction to Ayurveda. Although it is promoted as a weight loss book, it focuses on the relationship between our gut lining, the blood brain barrier, and our mental and physical health.

Dr. Chaudhary is a charismatic speaker. She is also an experienced doctor and researcher, and has participated in over twenty clinical research studies in the areas of multiple sclerosis, Alzheimer's disease, Parkinson's disease, ALS, and diabetic peripheral neuropathy.

The Prime begins with a charming description of her early life in India and describes her close relationship with her grandfather, who was a doctor and who ultimately inspired her to graduate from medical school with honors in psychiatry, and complete her neurology residency. Dr. Chaudhary's own health problems began when her family moved to America, and worsened when she entered medical school. A visiting Ayurvedic doctor told her that her headaches were due to problems in her gut. Once she began to incorporate Ayurveda into her life, she found that her health improved. She was trained in Maharishi Ayurveda and learned Transcendental Meditation, both of which she now prescribes to her patients.

I remember a talk Dr. Chaudhary gave about curing one woman of depression. She explained that once she understood her patient's unique Ayurvedic constitution and its imbalance, she was able to use simple treatments to take the woman from a state of total despair to being a loving, active person again. At the end of the treatment program, the woman's family came to see Dr. Chaudhary and thanked her for bringing their mother back to them. This is only one example among many of the effectiveness of Ayurveda's natural integration into modern medical practice.

Dr. Chaudhary describes her program as "a diet in reverse." You begin by taking a quiz to determine your level of toxicity and inflammation and then you choose a particular detox treatment program according to your degree of toxicity.

Dr. Chaudhary calls the first stage of her program "Activate a Biochemical Shift." It involves adding four activities to the daily routine:

1. Morning begins with you making a tea of cumin, coriander, and fennel seeds, to sip throughout the day. This starts to detoxify and balance the body.

2. Every other night, take a mixture of ground flax seeds and psyllium husks to help add fiber and improve elimination.

3. As part of the elimination routine, also take an Ayurvedic herbal preparation called Triphala.

4. The final part of the routine is a raw silk glove massage that helps remove toxins and improves circulation.

Stage two of Dr. Chaudhary's program is called "Crush Cravings." It consists of taking potent Ayurvedic herbs as well as juice and broth to help curb your cravings. She encourages you to keep a Cravings Journal.

The third stage is "Ignite Energy and Fat." One of Dr. Chaudhary's main tools for detoxification and increasing digestive power is an Ayurvedic herbal preparation called guggul, made from the gum of the myrrh tree. She also suggests the addition of fat-burning curry powder to meals. Finally, she prescribes a traditional premeal Ayurvedic digestive aid, consisting of a mixture of fresh ginger juice, lemon juice, and salt.

Stage four is "Biohack Your Lifestyle Habits." This involves changes in your routine:

- Make lunch your main meal of the day

- No raw vegetables until your gut is stronger

- Avoid ice-cold drinks

- Learn to meditate

- Get to bed by 10 p.m. each night

The result of this program, Dr. Chaudhary explains, is not only weight loss but the rejuvenation of your entire digestive system, and the improvement of your overall mental and physical health. She explains that excess weight is a result of the body being in a toxic, inflammatory state and that if it is not prepared or "primed" for weight loss, you will be engaged in a physiological struggle. Dr. Chaudhary does not focus on the various foods you can't have, but on how to purify your body using simple herbs and teas.

Once you have gone through the detox program, however, it is important to know what foods are best for your unique constitution. Dr. Chaudhary has used her program to alleviate conditions such as Alzheimer's disease, diabetes, obesity, and coronary artery disease. She also extends the idea of Leaky Gut to a Leaky Brain and describes how Ayurveda can help correct both situations. She has appeared on *The Dr. Oz Show* many times and is able to convey complex information about both the gut and brain in a practical and easy-to-understand manner.

Gut Rap Q & A:

Ms. Natural: I enjoyed her book very much and I'm interested in the concept of mental toxins. Could you explain it more?

Doc Gut: Dr. Chaudhary tells us that mental toxins are like undigested emotions in our psyche, which might be the result of past trauma or unresolved problems. In Ayurveda, there is no distinction between toxins in the body and toxins in the mind.

H Bomb: If the digestive system is constantly shedding its cells every few days and replacing them with new ones, why is detox even necessary?

Doc Gut: According to Dr. Chaudhary, detox is a normal part of the body's functioning. Our liver and kidneys detox all the time. If the gut bacteria are imbalanced, then the newly developed cells in the gut will be disrupted by an ever-growing population of harmful bacteria. We must remove the causes of the problem, which include a poor diet, weak digestion, a disrupted gut bacteria, and the accumulation of toxins.

Ms. Natural: I've heard that people can feel tired when toxins are coming out.

Doc Gut: That's very true. Dr. Chaudhary explains that toxins can produce lethargy in the body while they are leaving.

Ms. Natural: Why don't other doctors agree with all this?

Doc Gut: Dr. Chaudhary says that conventional doctors are following what they learned in medical school. As a doctor in the field of Integrative Medicine, she is looking at the latest data from cutting-edge research and combining these findings with the time-tested knowledge from traditional medicine.

Ms. Natural: Does she talk about food addiction?

Doc Gut: Dr. Chaudhary explains that the brain has a remarkable ability to adapt to what is going on in your body. If you eat a lot of sugar, the brain adapts. If you exercise daily, the brain adapts. She gives an example of drug dependence in which the process of neuroadaptation can work against us. Science has shown that many illegal drugs cause the release of the neurotransmitter dopamine in specific reward centers in the brain. Dopamine results in the feeling of pleasure. If enough drugs are taken, the brain adapts by reducing the number of dopamine receptors. The unfortunate end result is that more and more drugs must be taken to produce the same effects and the person gradually becomes addicted. If they stop using the drug, there are terrible withdrawal symptoms and a vicious cycle is created.

If we apply these same principles to eating sugary foods, we can see where it leads. First, we become addicted; then we start to gain weight and reach an obese state, which results in health problems like diabetes or cardiovascular disease. The good news is that if we detoxify and change our diet for a long enough period, our brain will adapt and return to a normal healthy state.

REFERENCES:

The Prime: Prepare and Repair Your Body for Spontaneous Weight Loss by Dr. Kulreet Chaudhary, Harmony, 2016

Braniste, V et al., The gut microbiota influences blood-brain barrier permeability in mice. *Science translational medicine* 2014; 6(263):263ra158

Diana, M, The Dopamine Hypothesis of Drug Addiction and Its Potential Therapeutic Value. *Frontiers in Psychiatry* 2011; 2:64

CHAPTER 26

Gut

Of all the books on the gut, the simplest and most charming is *Gut* by Giulia Enders. Giulia had not yet finished her doctorate when she wrote the book, and yet a million copies were sold in Germany alone. She kindly gives part of the credit to her sister, whose quirky clear illustrations complement her easy and informative writing style.

Beginning with the basics, she explains each part of the digestive system, with easily understood examples. Giulia describes how various types of food are digested and where they are absorbed into our gut. She includes all the hot topics—gluten intolerance, lactose intolerance, and Poopology 101. Yes, she describes everything we ever wondered about the different shapes and types of poop, feces, or stool—whatever we want to call it.

Ancient Chinese court physicians used to examine the poop of the Emperor every day. This tradition is also found in other countries. Giulia explains that the color, consistency, and smell of feces all tell us something specific about a person's health.

Let's consider color. Stool colors can range from light brown to yellow-brown to dark brown because of the presence of red blood cells. Our body makes and destroys over 2 million red blood cells each day. Giulia explains that when the red blood cells break down, their red pigment first turns green, and then yellow. Some of this pigment goes into the urine and makes it yellow. The rest of the pigment goes to the liver, and then to the lower gut, where the bacteria turn it brown.

If the color of the stool is between light brown and yellow, it can be the result of a harmless condition called Gilbert's syndrome, in which the mechanism for the breakdown of red blood cells isn't working properly. This condition affects about 8% of the world's population, and its only known disadvantage is that these people cannot tolerate the drug acetaminophen as well as others.

If a person has taken antibiotics or had some infection, the color of their poop may be yellowish since the gut bacteria are disrupted and unable to turn the red blood cell pigment to its normal brown color.

Gray or light brown poop can indicate serious conditions in which there may be a kink in the tube between the liver and gut, preventing the broken down blood pigment from making its way to the gut.

Very dark, black, or red poop may mean that there are blood cells in the poop, which could be due to several things. If it is bright red, this could be due to hemorrhoids. If it is dark red or black, it could be something more severe, like an ulcer. We learn about one exception—if we eat beets, our urine and poop will have a reddish color.

Giulia also talks about a diagnostic medical observation procedure, called the Bristol scale, which divides the consistency of poop into seven main types. Type 1, for example, is defined as separate hard lumps, which indicate constipation. Type 4 is described as soft sausage shaped poop, which is healthy. Type 7 is liquid poop or diarrhea, which could indicate anything from a simple bacterial infection to IBS.

This type of classification also tells the doctor how long it has taken for indigestible particles to pass through the patient's gut. Type 1 can take 100 hours, showing serious constipation. Type 7 indicates that the complete digestion of a meal took about 10 hours. A further consideration is how quickly the poop sinks in the toilet bowl. Healthy poop sinks slowly, while constipated poop which is denser sinks quickly.

Most people believe that poop is made up of the food we have eaten, but this is not the case. Its composition is three-quarters water. The lower intestine has a remarkable capacity to reabsorb water and minerals, which would otherwise leave the body as waste; however, some water remains in the poop, so that it's soft enough to exit easily. The remaining solids may be divided into three parts: gut bacteria that are no longer needed in the large intestine, undigested fibrous material, and a mixture of waste products, which can include anything from food coloring to cholesterol.

In the last part of her book, Giulia dives into the world of microbes, giving us detailed descriptions of different kinds of bacteria. In tune with her audience, she understands what questions might be on our minds, and addresses each one carefully and humorously.

Her explanations describe the digestive system, as well as the immune and nervous systems, and how each interacts with the gut bacteria. If your understanding of physiology is limited and you need to catch up on the basics, this book is for you. If you want the real scoop about food allergies, or you would like to learn more about probiotics and prebiotics, it's all in this book.

The book's only flaw is one that plagues all books in this field. New knowledge is unfolding so fast that it's impossible to include the latest findings because they change, literally every day.

Gut Rap Q & A:

H Bomb: I've heard that our appendix is just a useless part of our digestive tract. What does Giulia say?

Doctor Gut: She maintains that it's an important part, which has been overlooked simply because of the lack of knowledge about gut bacteria. She describes the appendix as resembling a deflated balloon we might find at a children's party. It is located between the small intestine and large intestine, and off to the side where food particles don't normally pass, making it unsuitable for digesting or absorbing food. This placement, however, is excellent for monitoring foreign microbes. The appendix consists almost completely of immune cells that help destroy harmful bacteria. It also acts as a storehouse for good bacteria, so if an unwanted bout of diarrhea comes tearing through our bowels, our appendix can replenish the gut with good bacteria.

Ms. Natural: What are the other kinds of poop besides Types 1, 4, and 7?

Doctor Gut: According to the Bristol scale, Type 2 is sausage shaped but lumpy, Type 3 is like a sausage but with cracks, Type 5 is soft with clear edges, and Type 6 is a mushy stool with ragged edges.

H Bomb: What more is there to say about poop?

Doctor Gut: A lot more. In the beginning of her book, Giulia asks: How Does Pooping Work? And Why That's An Important Question. She goes on to explain that our bodies have developed special mechanisms to help us eliminate properly. We have several different sphincters (rings of muscles): an outer one, which we can easily control, and an inner one to make sure everything is okay on the inside. There are also gas sensors between the two sphincters to make sure that gas pressure doesn't go too high, so that we occasionally ease out some wind when no one will notice.

Ms. Natural: Does Giulia consider other parts of the digestive system?

Doctor Gut: Beginning with the mouth, Giulia describes our digestive system from one end to the other using her sister's entertaining graphics and little-known facts. For example, she tells us that our saliva contains a painkiller stronger than morphine, which was only discovered in 2006. We produce very small amounts, but it helps ease sensitivity to different foods, or sores in the mouth. Our saliva also produces antibacterial substances. Since we don't produce much saliva at night, it's good that we make a habit of brushing our teeth before bed.

Ms. Natural: What does she say about sugar?

Doc Gut: A lot! She explains that if we eat table sugar, it enters our bloodstream very quickly. Even white bread is rapidly broken down into sugar, but wholegrain bread takes longer to digest and, therefore, our sugar levels don't rise as quickly. She tells us that a sugar rush makes our body do a lot of work, pumping out hormones, especially insulin, which can result in a tired feeling after the sugar explosion. She points out that never before has mankind consumed so much sugar, especially fructose, which is now part of most processed foods in the form of high fructose corn syrup. She doesn't advocate total abstinence, just moderation.

To illustrate how food is digested, she follows the digestion of a piece of cake from fork to toilet. She explains that there are faster guts that can do it in eight hours, and slower ones, which can take three and a half days!

Ms. Natural: What does she say about bacteria?

Doctor Gut: A third of this book is on bacteria. Giulia says that more than 95% of the world's bacteria are harmless to humans, and that we only began to get an overview of all the microorganisms in our body around 2007. It turns out that 99% of all the microorganisms in or on our body are located in our gut, and have an average total weight of about four and a half pounds for the normal person. The balance between good and bad bacteria is critical. She also goes into detail about the benefits of probiotics and prebiotics.

One of her humorous ideas was to post a picture of our favorite meal on "Facebug" (Facebook beware), which would immediately receive millions of likes and dislikes from bacteria friends.

REFERENCE:

Gut: The Inside Story of the Our Body's Most Underrated Organ by Giulia Enders, Greystone Books, 2015

Lewis, SJ and Heaton, KW, Stool Form Scale as a Useful Guide to Intestinal Transit Time. *Scan J Gastroenterol* 1997; 32 (9), 920-294

Varea, V et al., Malabsorption of carbohydrates and depression in children and adolescents. *J Pediatr Gastroenterol Nutr* 2005; 40(5):561-5

CHAPTER 27

I Contain Multitudes

An eloquent and compelling book on gut bacteria is *I Contain Multitudes* by Ed Yong. Beautifully written, it is filled with wonderful stories about strange animals and their relationship with even stranger bacteria.

Yong's favorite bacteria is *Wolbachia pipientis.* The most successful bacteria in the world, it infects half of all insects, spiders, scorpions, and similar creatures. He describes exciting research on *Wolbachia*, which suggests its potential to eliminate dengue fever. Dengue fever infects as many as 400 million people every year, killing tens of thousands. Up to now, there has been nothing anyone could do to either prevent or cure it, though it has long been known to be transmitted by a virus in the mosquito *Aedes aegypti.*

Over thirty years ago, Professor Scott O'Neill from Australia began research on how to eradicate dengue fever by using *Wolbachia*. An important breakthrough occurred in 2006 when one of his graduate students was able to insert a strain of *Wolbachia* into *Aedes aegypti.* The *Wolbachia* stopped the virus that causes dengue fever from reproducing, creating a new dynasty of dengue-free mosquitoes.

To test his research, O'Neill convinced residents of two areas in Australia to release hundreds of thousands of the dengue-free mosquitoes. In only a few months, *Wolbachia* had infected the entire mosquito population and virtually eliminated the chances of people ever being infected with dengue fever virus in those areas. The next step is to introduce the *Wolbachia*-infected mosquito into countries like Brazil, Indonesia, and Vietnam, where dengue is a far more severe problem.

Stopping insects from spreading a deadly human disease without using insecticides or genetic engineering is both novel and effective. And this is only the beginning of this research because mosquitoes also carry diseases like malaria and *Zika*, among others. The possibilities are unlimited. No wonder *Wolbachia* is Yong's favorite bacteria.

I Contain Multitudes also discusses the latest research on probiotics and fecal transplant. Yong explains that commercially available probiotics are not very effective because they mostly contain *Lactobacillus* and *Bifidobacterium*, which are present in such small quantities in most adults that they have no significant outcome in the restoration of the ecology of the gut bacteria. *Lactobacillus* and *Bifidobacterium* may offer some help for digestion, but will not, according to his opinion, remedy serious disease.

Doctors and scientists don't yet know which probiotics to use to cure specific diseases. They could try less well-known bacteria such as *Akkermansia muciniphilia*, whose presence in the gut correlates with a lower risk of obesity; however, *Akkermansia* has been found to be common in colorectal cancer patients.

We should note that diet is at least as important as the types and amounts of bacteria used in a probiotic because no bacteria can survive and establish itself unless it is fed the right food.

Bacteroides fragilis and *Faecalibacterium prausnitzii* are both associated with the anti-inflammatory action of the immune system and may be helpful in dealing with inflammatory bowel disease. *F. prausnitzii* has a much larger presence in the gut than *Lactobacillus*. In healthy adults, 1 out of every 20 bacteria are *F. prausnitzii*, so if it were part of a probiotic, it might have a better chance at making a lasting contribution. But this has yet to be proven.

Yong also gives two examples of research programs that tested the potential use of gut bacteria, one successful, the other not. One involved the bacteria *Synergistes jonesii*, named after the researcher Raymond Jones, who first discovered it in Hawaiian goats. Jones noticed that the goats were able to consume quantities of the toxic shrub *Leucaena,* with no ill effects. He hypothesized that *Synergistes jonesii* would enable livestock in Australia to also eat the *Leucaena.* Jones transported the bacteria from the goats in Hawaii to livestock in Australia, and his experiment worked. From then on, the Australian animals had a cheap and plentiful source of food that had previously been inedible.

The other example involved the bacteria *Oxalobacter formigenes,* a bacteria that digests the chemical oxalate as its only source of energy. Oxalate is present in plentiful amounts in foods like asparagus, beetroot, and spinach. When too much oxalate is consumed, it can both prevent the body from absorbing calcium and cause kidney stones. So it seemed like a great idea to consume *Oxalobacter* as a probiotic in order to prevent the formation of kidney stones. When tried experimentally, however, it didn't work. We don't even know why, only that it was not able to prevent kidney stones.

Why does one bacteria work and another doesn't? There are many factors involved. For one thing, the bacteria in our gut exists as a community, a complex network of codependency with one bacteria helping another. Maybe, Yong suggests, *Oxalobacter* needs a friend to keep it alive.

Fecal transplant has been proven to be far more successful than any probiotic formula. Yong calls a fecal transplant "an ecosystem transplant." We are not receiving 1 or 10 insignificant bacteria that have little chance of surviving; we're getting an entire community, which we already know can survive successfully in the gut.

Should fecal transplant be used to treat every digestive disease? Yong explains that fecal transplant is perfect for the *C. difficile* infection. Most patients with this type of infection ironically get it after taking too many antibiotics, which have decimated the patient's balance of friendly gut bacteria. When the person receives a fecal transplant, the new bacteria have no trouble recolonizing the gut and are able to dominate *C. difficile,* and repopulate without much resistance. In other diseases, it may be harder for the fecal transplant to reboot the entire system.

Yong reminds us that fecal transplant may be one of the least attractive treatments ever invented. Also, we don't know yet if there are side effects. Yong explains that most scientists do not see fecal transplant as a lasting solution. What they hope is that they will at some point be able to replace fecal transplant with a probiotic formula, which can then be supported by a diet that allows the new therapeutic bacteria to make a stronghold in the gut and thrive.

Yong also makes the very important point that one size may not fit all. By this, he means that we may have to personalize the probiotic formula for each individual. He gives an example of the drug digoxin, which is derived from the plant foxglove and is used to help patients with a failing heart. The drug usually makes the heart beat stronger and with a slower and more regular beat. However, in 1 out of 10 patients, the drug doesn't do this because of the presence of a type of bacteria called *Eggerthella lenta*, which has the strange ability to render digoxin medically useless.

Yong predicts that the future of modern medicine lies in microbiome medicine. It may not be long before all diseases are diagnosed and treated through a more complete understanding of the state of our gut bacteria.

I highly recommend Ed Yong's book for anyone who loves both science and literature, and who wants to dive deeper into the symbiotic relationship between bacteria and animals.

Gut Rap Q & A:

Ms. Natural: Can you give us some other examples of symbiotic relationships?

Doc Gut: The book is filled with wonderful stories, for example, the relationship between the Hawaiian Bobtail Squid and a luminous bacteria called *Vibro fisheri*. The squid is the size of a golf ball and carries the bacteria in two chambers on its underside. When the squid moves in the water, light emanating from the bacteria closely resembles moonlight and hides the squid's silhouette from beneath. This is a protective mechanism, which shields it from predators. As Ed Yong writes, "This animal casts no shadow."

Even more remarkable is how the Hawaiian Bobtail Squid gives *Vibro fisheri* exclusive housing rights, excluding all other bacteria. It does this by producing an antimicrobial substance, which is neutral to *Vibro fisheri* but repellent to other bacteria. The squid also allows this bacteria to make its way into its inner chambers, becoming an elite club *of one*. In exchange for this exclusive residence, *Vibro fisheri* fuels the light mechanism that protects the squid for the rest of its life. This is the ultimate symbiotic relationship: *Mi casa es su casa—My home is your home.*

One other example is the petite flatworm *Paracatenula*, which lives in ocean floor sediments around the world. Half of its body contains friendly bacteria, which help provide energy for the flatworm, and even act as a battery that stores energy in certain compounds. What is fascinating is that these bacteria, and the energy they store, are what allow the flatworm to regenerate. It can be cut into two pieces or more, and each piece will regenerate to create a whole worm as long as there are enough bacteria preserved in the segment.

H Bomb: How do bacteria interfere with medicine?

Doc Gut: Yong cites a number of drugs that are affected by our gut bacteria. Sulfasalazine, for example, is a drug used to treat rheumatoid arthritis and IBD, but it only works when the right gut bacteria convert it into an active state. Another drug called Irinotecan, which is used to treat colon cancer, can be adversely affected by certain gut bacteria to create bad side effects.

H Bomb: You describe the bacteria *Wolbachia* as if it's some kind of savior of mankind, but from what I've read, it's the insect scourge of the world!

Doc Gut: That's an excellent observation. *Wolbachia's* primary concern is to perpetuate itself by infecting insects and being passed on to their offspring. However, it can only be passed to the next generation via females. As a result, it may inadvertently reduce the male insect population and expand the female portion. In wasps, for example, *Wolbachia* alters the reproductive mechanisms in the females so that they reproduce asexually through cloning. The males are no longer necessary for reproduction.

There are many other examples of how *Wolbachia* reduces the male population. In the case of the blue-moon butterfly, *Wolbachia* kills the male embryo. In woodlice, it impedes the creation of male hormones and turns males into females. These are only a few of its many tricks.

REFERENCE:

I Contain Multitudes: The Microbes Within Us and a Grander View of Life by Ed Yong, Ecco, 2016

Walker, T et al., The wMel Wolbachia strain blocks dengue and invades caged Aedes aegypti populations. *Nature* 2011; 476,450-453

McGraw, EA and O'Neil, SL, Beyond insecticides: new thinking on an ancient problem. *Nat Rev Microbiol* 2013; 11, 181-193

CHAPTER 28

Eat Dirt

One of the most popular experts in the field of gut repair is Dr. Josh Axe, whose new book is *Eat Dirt: Why Leaky Gut May Be the Root Cause of Your Health Problems and 5 Surprising Steps to Cure It*. Dr. Axe challenges modern beliefs about hygiene and provides practical solutions as well as the latest research findings on gut repair. His basic premise is that the source of most disease is a leaky gut. Clear and easy to read, with excellent graphics, the book explains the science behind Leaky Gut Syndrome and the steps you can take to heal it.

Dr. Axe's basic five-step program is easy to remember:

- Remove
- Reseed
- Restore
- Release
- Reseal

The first step is to eliminate foods that damage your gut health, including: wheat and other grains, commercial cow's milk, sugar, hydrogenated oils, GMO foods, and the toxic chemicals commonly found in processed food and beverages. All of these, according to Dr. Axe, have bad effects, such as destroying beneficial gut bacteria, feeding harmful bacteria, and damaging the intestinal wall. The result is leaky gut and ultimately chronic inflammation.

The second step is to reseed your gut with "good dirt" and soil based probiotic supplements. He goes into detail to help you find acceptable ways of eating dirt!

The third step is to restore the gut by beginning a bone broth fast for three days, and then eating good food: organic fruits, vegetables, meats, nuts, raw cultured dairy products, fermented vegetables, fermented beverages, coconut products, wild-caught salmon, sprouted seeds, and high-fiber foods that act as prebiotics.

The fourth step is to release and reduce emotional stress: have a massage or reflexology treatment, do something active, drink a warm glass of chamomile tea, read something uplifting, use essential oils, try a magnesium supplement, listen to music, and go "forest bathing," which can be as simple as a walk in the woods.

The fifth step involves resealing the leaky gut through probiotics, digestive enzymes, L-glutamine, licorice root, collagen, frankincense, and other supplements.

Eat Dirt contains an amazing amount of useful information ranging from how to choose the best probiotics to why we should eat organic non-GMO food. There's also an extensive section on essential oils and how they can heal your body and mind. Dr. Axe explains why it's so important to use the highest quality essential oils derived from organically grown plants.

The book has several quizzes, but the most interesting one helps you determine your gut type. Dr. Axe introduces five gut types based on Traditional Chinese Medicine: Candida Gut, Stressed Gut, Immune Gut, Gastric Gut, and Toxic Gut.

The Candida Gut Type, for example, is characterized by an overgrowth of *Candida albicans*, the most common type of yeast infection. In Chinese medicine, this type is related to the concept of dampness or an accumulation of fluids in the body. *Candida* thrives in a damp environment. The three organs that suffer the most from this condition are the spleen, pancreas, and small intestine. Dr. Axe's program includes the elimination of foods that are toxic to the spleen and small intestine, along with the consumption of therapeutic foods and supplements, and changes in your lifestyle and daily routine.

Eat Dirt ends with a section that provides specific tips on how to transform your home and diet to heal your gut. This very comprehensive book provides many interesting case studies and practical programs, and an extensive list of scientific references.

Gut Rap Q & A:

H Bomb: Tell me about the Toxic Gut Type.

Doc Gut: This type of gut has problems with the liver and gallbladder.

H Bomb: I had gallstones so maybe that relates to me.

Doc Gut: Dr. Axe explains that most gallstones are formed as a result of the body's bile becoming supersaturated with cholesterol. This can also happen due to a slower moving gut, obesity, and high-fat diets. Traditional Chinese Medicine attributes problems of the liver to emotions of anger, frustration, and lack of forgiveness.

I'm not assuming that you experience these emotions, I'm just stating what the author says.

H Bomb: I get it, Doc.

Doc Gut: According to Chinese medicine, the Toxic Gut involves the wood element and relates to the spring season when things are beginning to grow. Dr. Axe recommends eating green vegetables and fruits, which are full of enzymes that are good for your gall-bladder. He also recommends dandelion tea or milk thistle tea, as well as making a list of people you need to forgive.

H Bomb: Okay Doc, let's move on to another type.

Doc Gut: There's the Gastric Type, which often suffers from acid reflux or indigestion, and a condition we talked about earlier, small intestinal bacteria overgrowth or SIBO. According to Chinese medicine, the organs involved with this gut type are the stomach, spleen, and pancreas. The person tends to have a fiery personality. The main causes of a gastric gut are low stomach acid, the overuse of antacids, insufficient chewing, and overeating. Again, Dr. Axe has a whole program to cure it.

Ms. Natural: Could you talk about the final two types?

Doc Gut: The symptoms of the Immune Gut usually indicate a severe form of leaky gut, which can lead to autoimmune conditions such as inflammatory bowel disease. The diet in this program is aimed at reducing immune reactions and giving the gut easy-to-digest food. Bone broth is valuable for this type. According to Chinese medicine, the individuals most susceptible to this kind of gut disorder are those who tend to have an emotional response to conflict that involves either insecurity, grief, or lack of confidence.

Ms. Natural: And the Stressed Gut?

Doc Gut: The Stressed Gut is common in people who overreact to stress. This might be a strong willed type A personality who is often uncompromising. Improving their reaction to stress is very important. Dr. Axe focuses on the adrenal glands, which release hormones involved in stress reactions. Such individuals need a diet and lifestyle that calms the adrenal glands and repairs the gut. One simple piece of advice is to avoid caffeine and alcohol.

Ms. Natural: What tips does he have for improving the home?

Doc Gut: He gives instructions on how to make items like home-made house cleaners, laundry soap, and probiotic toothpaste.

Ms. Natural: Does he say anything about Teflon pots and pans?

Doc Gut: He calls them time savers that could be killing us. He strongly suggests looking at the Environmental Working Group website to learn about removing toxicity from your home and gaining a better understanding about what home products can be hazardous to your health.

REFERENCES:

Eat Dirt: Why Leaky Gut May Be the Root Cause of Your Health Problems and 5 Surprising Steps to Cure It by Dr. Josh Axe, Harper Wave, 2016

Li, X and Atkinson, MA, The role of gut permeability in the pathogenesis of type 1 diabetes—a solid or leaky concept? *Pediatr Diabetes* 2015; 7, 485-92

Fasano, A, Intestinal permeability and its regulation by zonulin: diagnosis and therapeutic implications. *Clin Gastroenterol Hepatol* 2012; 10,1096-100

CHAPTER 29

Fat for Fuel

Perhaps the biggest name in alternative health is Dr. Joseph Mercola. For years he has dominated this world with his books and an information-packed website that has 15 million unique visitors and 40 million page views a month. His latest book is *Fat for Fuel: A Revolutionary Diet to Combat Cancer, Boost Brain Power, and Increase Your Energy.*

In this book, Dr. Mercola explains what first inspired him to turn to a more holistic approach to health. In 1995, he attended a series of lectures by Dr. Ron Rosedale, who explained the importance of controlling high insulin levels to prevent the occurrence of chronic disorders such as diabetes, obesity, and heart disease. Dr. Mercola reveals that this was the moment he realized the need to minimize pharmaceutical solutions with all their side effects, and focus on natural treatments based on diet.

An early book, *The No-Grain Diet: Conquer Carbohydrate Addiction and Stay Slim for Life,* was one of the first *New York Times* best sellers to advocate limiting refined carbohydrates and processed food. And in his book *Sweet Deception: Why Splenda,*

NutraSweet, and the FDA May Be Hazardous to Your Health, he was again one of the first doctors to speak openly about the dangers of artificial sweeteners. Dr. Mercola constantly goes up against the FDA and big business in his crusade to improve our health habits.

After treating more than 25,000 patients, his focus is on the importance of eating high quality fats and activating the body's natural ability to burn fat as a primary fuel rather than glucose. *Fat for Fuel* challenges the current scientific opinion that cancer is a genetic disease caused by chromosomal damage. Dr. Mercola cites research that indicates that it is caused by defective metabolic processes in our mitochondria.

The mitochondria are the energy engines of our body. There are thousands in every cell and they generate 90% of the energy necessary to stay alive and well. According to Dr. Mercola, when the mitochondria become damaged in large numbers, it's impossible to stay healthy.

Dr. Mercola explains that our food choices have a direct impact on our mitochondria. With the right food, the genetic material in the mitochondria is far less likely to become damaged and trigger a chain reaction that can lead to cancer. He advocates a ketogenic diet, low in carbohydrates and high in healthy fats, and refers to his diet program, which helps the mitochondria stay healthy, as Mitochondrial Metabolic Therapy (MMT).

Fat for Fuel provides an excellent history of the tragic misunderstanding of the effects of fats on our health. It began with an American researcher, Ancel Keys, who was on the cover of *Time* magazine in 1961 and hailed as the most influential nutrition expert. His most important study, the Seven Countries Study, was published in 1970 and has been cited by numerous other studies.

Dr. Mercola points out that this study never proved causation, only association, between saturated fats and heart disease. Despite this serious flaw, Ancel Keys was able to gain wide acceptance by the American medical community. In 1977, the US released the first national dietary guidelines, which promoted cutting back on fat intake and eating more grains. It also recommended replacing natural animal fats with processed vegetable oils. According to Dr. Mercola, the result is that for over fifty years we have been following incorrect medical advice about the effect of fats and causing untold damage to our health. The war on fat continues to this day with enormous consequences.

Dr. Mercola reviews all the latest studies, which indicate that there is no difference in the risks of heart disease and stroke between people with the lowest and the highest intakes of fat.

The book goes on to describe the benefits of Mitochondrial Metabolic Therapy, clarifying many issues about protein intake. Dr. Mercola shows why his diet is an important refinement over the Paleo diet. *Fat for Fuel* is filled with the easiest possible explanations of complex and hard to understand biochemical pathways that underlie every metabolic process in our body.

He concludes by explaining that it is time to reverse the demonization of healthy fats and teach our body how to use them as a primary fuel. In this way, we can lose weight, reduce inflammation, and prevent and cure chronic disease. He cautions, however, that improving mitochondrial function is an evolving science and will take many years to be widely accepted.

Gut Rap Q & A:

Ms. Natural: What does Dr. Mercola say about protein?

Doc Gut: He says that both the Atkins and Paleo diets have been misinterpreted by people who have placed great emphasis on protein. He says that the original diet programs included recommendations for more green leafy vegetables but somehow these got lost. He adds that Americans eat too much protein, and specifically warns against meat proteins that have too much of the amino acid methionine. He says that we don't want to eliminate this amino acid, but we do want to lower it.

Ms. Natural: What does he say about calorie restriction? I heard that it's been shown to slow down the aging process.

Doc Gut: Dr. Mercola explains that in many animal studies, lowering caloric intake has been shown to slow the aging process. This type of diet alters the expression of hundreds to thousands of genes. He claims that his own MMT diet of high-fat, adequate-protein, and low-carbs, has a similar effect, but without feelings of deprivation.

Ms. Natural: Does he say anything else about preventing aging?

Doc Gut: He mentions that insulin is an important factor. If our body has enough food, insulin sends a signal to reproduce. If our body perceives that there is not enough food, it turns on protective and regenerative mechanisms to ensure survival through the tough times. Dr. Mercola tells us that we have a better chance of living longer if we have lower insulin levels.

One of the factors that keeps insulin high, according to Dr. Mercola, is excess protein, which stimulates the production of a particular hormone known as insulin-like-growth factor or IGF-1. This hormone tells the body to grow by sending a message for the cells to reproduce, which costs the body extra energy. Studies show that animals that produce less IGF-1 live longer.

He recounts a fascinating study of a community living in a distant corner of Ecuador, who are afflicted with a rare form of dwarfism called Laron syndrome. This genetic condition causes them to make less IGF-1 and as a result, they live longer and have almost no cases of diabetes or cancer.

H Bomb: I heard that Dr. Mercola doesn't like people taking too many antioxidants. What's with that? I take a boatload.

Doc Gut: He has an interesting perspective. He says that if we take too many antioxidant supplements, it may stop cancer cells from turning on a built in mechanism that causes them to self-destruct. He advocates taking antioxidants, but not by the boatload.

Ms. Natural: What are his other books about?

Doc Gut: They cover many different topics, from children's diets to sunlight exposure to the "next big pandemic." A number of his books are listed below.

REFERENCES:

Fat for Fuel: A Revolutionary Diet to Combat Cancer, Boost Brain Power, and Increase Your Energy by Dr. Joseph Mercola, Hay House, Inc.; 1 edition, May 16, 2017

Effortless Healing: 9 Simple Ways to Sidestep Illness, Shed Excess Weight, and Help Your Body Fix Itself by Dr. Joseph Mercola (Author), David Perlmutter (Foreword), Harmony; 1 edition, February 24, 2015

Dr. Mercola's Total Health Cookbook & Program: 150 Delicious Grain-Free Recipes & Proven Metabolic Type Plan to Prevent Disease, Optimize Weight and Live Longer by Dr. Joseph Mercola, Mercola.com; 14017th edition, 1994

The No-Grain Diet: Conquer Carbohydrate Addiction and Stay Slim for Life by Joseph Mercola, Alison Rose Levy, Plume; Reprint edition, March 30, 2004

Take Control of Your Health by Joseph Mercola, Kendra Pearsall, Mercola.com, 2007

Sweet Deception: Why Splenda, NutraSweet, and the FDA May Be Hazardous to Your Health by Dr. Joseph Mercola, Dr. Kendra Degen Pearsall, Thomas Nelson; 1 edition, November 7, 2006

Generation XL: Raising Healthy, Intelligent Kids in a High-Tech, Junk-Food World by Dr. Joseph Mercola, Dr. Ben Lerner, Thomas Nelson; 1 edition, March 20, 2007

The Great Bird Flu Hoax: The Truth They Don't Want You to Know About the "Next Big Pandemic" by Dr. Joseph Mercola, Thomas Nelson; 1 edition, September 19, 2006

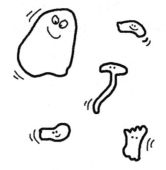

PART 5

PAST AND FUTURE

CHAPTER 30

Traditional Medicine

Food is regarded as medicine in all systems of traditional or natural medicine. One of the oldest systems, Ayurveda, which originated in India many thousands of years ago, has a number of concepts that I found difficult to translate into modern scientific terms. But the latest research on gut bacteria has made it far easier to understand these ancient ideas.

Ayurveda is very clear that if our food is not properly broken down and digested, the result is the production of a substance referred to as *ama*. Once ama builds up in the body, disease follows. It's hard for us, as Westerners, to pin down exactly what ama is. Is it undigested food, is it bacteria, or is it a type of toxin?

Let's try to understand ama from the perspective of the gut bacteria. What happens to the gut wall when the gut bacteria become disrupted? Most health experts now agree that the gut wall starts to break down, resulting in a situation, which is either called increased intestinal permeability or Leaky Gut Syndrome. In this condition undigested food, unfriendly bacteria, and environmental toxins, enter the bloodstream. This is an excellent description

227

of the ancient concept of the presence and accumulation of ama in the body. The word ama does not designate a single substance; rather it defines numerous substances or toxins that get into the body and set off the immune system, creating health problems and disease.

Another term, which is a little less difficult to understand, is *agni*. In Ayurveda, agni means the fire of digestion. In modern medicine, we might equate agni with the digestive enzymes that break down different types of foods. This is a fairly straightforward explanation, which we can now extend to include the digestive power of bacteria in our lower gut. We know that some food doesn't get digested in the small intestine, where digestive enzymes are most abundant, but proceeds to the large intestine, where our food is digested and fermented by bacteria. The sensitivity of our gut and the types of bacteria present, are what determine how much gas is produced, and whether we experience proper digestion or bloating, pain, constipation, or diarrhea.

All of these symptoms are significant considerations in Ayurveda and are much easier to understand if we include the latest information about the gut bacteria.

Another complex concept in Ayurveda has to do with three basic qualities in the body. These are called Vata, Pitta, and Kapha. They are not easily translated into modern science but Vata refers to all the systems of the body that control movement, including the nervous system. Pitta refers to the systems of the body concerned with metabolism, such as the digestive system. Kapha refers to

228

those systems involved with structure and lubrication, such as the bones and joints.

Each person has a unique combination of Vata, Pitta, and Kapha. In previous books, we have called this our Brain/Body Nature since it involves a mixture of mental and physical characteristics. In this book, however, we talk about our Gut/Brain Nature.

There are many interesting correlations between the balance of gut bacteria and the different kinds of Ayurvedic natures. In Ayurveda, the seat of Vata is in the colon and Vata disorders are said to make up 80% of all diseases. The ancient healers realized that all diseases, even those of the nervous system, begin in the gut.

One of the most well-studied medicinal plants in the Ayurvedic tradition is turmeric, and its active ingredient, curcumin. It is estimated that turmeric and curcumin have been the subject of over 5000 peer-reviewed and published biomedical studies, with 600 potential preventive and therapeutic applications, as well as 175 distinct beneficial physiological effects on such diseases as ulcerative colitis, stomach ulcers, osteoarthritis, heart disease, cancer, and neurodegenerative disorders. A number of recent studies also describe how turmeric interacts with the gut bacteria to modulate different aspects of the process of digestion.

In 2015, the Nobel Prize in medicine was awarded to Youyou Tu for her study of the effects of *Artemisia annua*, an herb from Traditional Chinese Medicine or TCM, that is now used as an effective treatment for malaria. TCM places a great deal of emphasis on the gut and the process of digestion and includes many procedures similar to those of Ayurveda to detoxify the gut and repair damage to its lining.

Natural medicine contains a wealth of time-tested procedures to improve the state of our gut and the state of our health. Meditation is an integral part of Ayurveda and its sister discipline, Yoga. I have studied the Transcendental Meditation (TM) program for over fifty years, and it has been shown to have many beneficial effects on mental and physical health. One of the latest studies published on TM reports a 48% reduction in heart attacks, strokes, and deaths in the TM group as compared to randomly matched controls. Over $25 million in grants from the National Institutes of Health have supported research on the beneficial effects of TM on cardiovascular disease.

The physiological changes during TM have been studied extensively and it is clear from this research that this particular meditation has a remarkable ability to reduce stress. We know that stress shuts down and totally disrupts the digestive process and there's little doubt that it is a major contributor to gut disorders and the imbalance of gut bacteria. I feel strongly that it is vital for science to explore how meditation affects gut bacteria.

I once asked a bright young group of medical students in South India whether they would be interested in learning to meditate if I could show strict scientific research on its benefits for health and longevity. To my surprise, only a handful expressed any curiosity at all. I wasn't sure why, so I took a different approach and asked how many of them would be interested if I were to offer a new pill, developed in our Western laboratories, which would have beneficial effects on their health and longevity. Virtually all the students raised their hands. They were more than willing to take this new pill. Granted, they were medical students, yet even more than others, they should have been aware of the negative side effects and shortcoming of pills. Why, then, were they so eager to take a pill rather than meditate?

I finally asked who would be interested if I could demonstrate that during meditation a new chemical was produced, one which was identical to the pill I had offered. This time, almost everyone's hand shot up. As long as I could explain the mechanics of meditation in terms of pills and chemicals, there was no prejudice or misconception.

What I was offering the students was not merely a fanciful idea. Laboratories around the world today are studying everything about meditation, from brain imaging to changes in neurotransmitters, to gene expression.

The ancient Vedic texts, including those of Ayurveda, refer to two interesting substances that were considered to be the body's natural mediators of ideal health and longevity. These substances are called *ojas* and *soma*. Ayurvedic texts describe ojas as the finest product of digestion, while soma is described as a plant, which has unique and remarkable properties for increasing awareness.

Maharishi Mahesh Yogi, the founder of the Transcendental Meditation technique, has explained that these words, ojas and soma, refer to the same substance, which is produced by a digestive system that is free from stress and a nervous system free from stress. He described this natural substance as the biochemical basis of the brain's ability to support higher and more comprehensive states of awareness. Soma is a product of our body's natural pharmacy, and is created by the interaction of a perfectly functioning nervous system and a perfectly functioning digestive system. If we are stressed, or if our digestion is not working properly, our body is not able to produce this natural substance.

I have always been excited by the prospect of identifying soma. With the new understanding of the gut bacteria and the gut-brain axis, science is in a much better position to carry out such an investigation. It is remarkable that these ancient concepts can now begin to be understood in modern scientific terms.

Gut Rap Q & A:

H Bomb: So you're telling us that we have to go to some cave in India for the answers to our gut health?

Doc Gut: No. There's a wealth of knowledge in the ancient systems of medicine that has been ignored because it is not expressed in the language of modern science. Each time a scientific study is published on practices from these traditional systems of medicine, it becomes easier for modern medicine to understand their value.

Ms. Natural: I have heard that Ayurveda defines 6 stages of disease.

Doc Gut: Yes, that's true. The first four of these stages have to do with the early development of disease and only the last two stages are recognized and used by modern medicine. By understanding more subtle aspects of the disease process, Ayurveda takes a preventive approach and restores balance to the physiology before disease can develop.

H-Bomb: What about organic food?

Doc Gut: Ayurveda and other systems of natural medicine strongly emphasize the quality of the food we eat and most alternative health practitioners recommend eating organic food to avoid pesticides. The danger of genetically modified food or GMOs is an area of great concern and many countries in the world ban them entirely. I include several excellent books on this important topic in the reference section at the end of the chapter.

Ms. Natural: How can I find out more about Ayurveda?

Doctor Gut: You will find more information about Ayurveda in later chapters and also at docgut.com and in the reference sections.

Ms. Natural: How do I learn TM?

Doc Gut: A useful book that answers all types of questions about TM is *An Introduction to Transcendental Meditation: Improve Your Brain Functioning, Create Ideal Health, and Gain Enlightenment Naturally, Easily, Effortlessly.* You'll find more information on the benefits of TM, as well as where to find a qualified teacher on tm.org and tmrefer.org.

REFERENCES:

Maharishi Ayurveda and Vedic Technology: Creating Ideal Health for the Individual and World, Adapted and Updated from The Physiology of Consciousness: Part 2 by Robert Keith Wallace, PhD, Dharma Publications, 2016

Dey, N et al., Regulators of gut motility revealed by a gnotobiotic model of diet-microbiome interactions related to traveling. *Cell* 2015; 163(1):95-107

Kashyap, P, Eat Your Curry. *Cell host & microbe* 2015; 18(4):385-387.

Seeds of Deception: Exposing Industry and Government Lies About the Safety of the Genetically Engineered Foods You're Eating by Jeffrey M. Smith, Yes Books, 2003

Altered Genes, Twisted Truth: How the Venture to Genetically Engineer Our Food Has Subverted Science, Corrupted Government, and Systematically Deceived the Public, 1st Edition, by Steven Druker, Clear River Press; 2015

An Introduction to Transcendental Meditation: Improve Your Brain Functioning, Create Ideal Health, and Gain Enlightenment Naturally, Easily, Effortlessly by Robert Keith Wallace, PhD, and Lincoln Akin Norton, Dharma Publications, 2016

Transcendental Meditation: A Scientist's Journey to Happiness, Health, and Peace, Adapted and Updated from The Physiology of Consciousness: Part 1 by Robert Keith Wallace, PhD, Dharma Publications, 2016

The Neurophysiology of Enlightenment: How the Transcendental Meditation and TM-Sidhi Program Transform the Functioning of the Human Body, by Robert Keith Wallace, PhD, Dharma Publications, 2016

Dharma Parenting: Understand your Child's Brilliant Brain for Greater Happiness, Health, Success, and Fulfillment by Robert Keith Wallace, PhD, and Fred Travis, PhD, Tarcher/Perigee, 2016

CHAPTER 31

The Future of Medicine

Integrative Medicine is one of many emerging fields in modern medicine. As its name implies, it consists of a complementary combination of traditional and modern treatment programs that deal with the health of the whole person. At our university, Maharishi University of Management, we offer a Master's degree in Maharishi Ayurveda and Integrative Medicine, which focuses on each of the eight major systems of the body, viewed from the perspective of both modern medicine and ancient health practices.

Lifestyle Medicine and Personalized Medicine are two new areas in modern medicine that incorporate diet, probiotics, prebiotics, exercise, behavior, and meditation. In Personalized Medicine, doctors use a person's genetic makeup to help tailor drug prescriptions and other treatment programs.

Microbiome Medicine is the most recent addition to these new fields that will rewrite much of what we know about the human body, as well as create a more comprehensive approach to healing that includes the world of microorganisms living in and around us. The mistaken and horribly misleading notion that we are separate from our environment must inevitably be replaced with the reality that we are part of it.

The first declaration of the World Health Organization's constitution asserts that: "Health is a state of complete physical, mental and social well-being and not merely the absence of disease or infirmity." The entire understanding of health must be redefined, with prevention at the forefront. Not surprisingly, some of the most specific and refined forms of health technology come from the oldest cultural traditions on earth, including Ayurveda and Chinese medicine.

Gut Rap Q & A:

H Bomb: What's the scientific proof for Ayurveda's constitutional analysis?

Doc Gut: Many research studies have been done on this topic. Some have looked at blood chemistry and physiological changes, while others have studied genetic expression to distinguish the main types or natures—Vata, Pitta, and Kapha. In one study, for example, total cholesterol, triglycerides, high LDL and low HDL concentrations—all common risk factors for cardiovascular disease—were reported to be higher in people with a Kapha nature compared to Pitta and Vata. Hemoglobin and red blood count were higher in Pittas compared to other types, and a pituitary hormone, prolactin, was shown to be higher in Vata natures.

Published studies on genetic expression have also been able to scientifically distinguish the three main natures. For instance, genes in the immune response pathways were turned on and more active in Pittas. Genes related to cell cycles were more active in Vatas, and genes in the immune signaling pathways were more active in Kaphas.

H Bomb: Why bother with all these different natures or types? Isn't it easier to just analyze a person's DNA and figure out what's needed?

Doc Gut: In principle, yes. In practice, no. Gene analysis is still at a crude state. While scientists have been able to map the human genome, it's very complicated to determine how genes are regulated. We have some 22,000 genes, and the information in them can be used in many different ways. There are a few cases in which a particular disease is caused by a mistake in a gene. In most cases, a chronic disease involves many different genes interacting in a highly complex manner.

Ms. Natural: What is Functional Medicine?

Doc Gut: According to the Institute for Functional Medicine, this field of medicine is a patient-centered approach, which addresses the whole person, rather than an isolated set of symptoms. In general, doctors spend more time with their patients, listening to their histories and considering the interactions among genetic, environmental, and lifestyle factors.

Ms. Natural: What's the difference between Functional Medicine and Integrative Medicine?

Doc Gut: The two fields are very much alike. Integrative medicine, as we have discussed, combines the best practices of modern medicine with those of traditional medicine, such as Traditional Chinese Medicine or Ayurveda. It makes use of vitamins, minerals, herbs, and homeopathy, among other treatments, and doctors can use modern tests, such as an MRI or blood analysis. They may also use newer tests that are not yet accepted by conventional physicians. In both cases, treatment programs emphasize changes in lifestyle that result in long-term improvement in health, rather than the short-term relief of symptoms through pills.

Ms. Natural: Is Integrative Medicine available in hospitals?

Doc Gut: There are Integrative Medicine Centers established in well-known hospitals and medical schools at Harvard, Stanford, Duke, University of Maryland, Northwestern, Ohio State, University of California at San Francisco, and the Mayo Clinic. Due to the efforts of a philanthropic organization called The Bravewell Collaborative, over the past two decades, a significant contribution has been made to the field of Integrative Medicine, with rapid growth in the number of clinical centers providing integrative medicine and medical schools teaching integrative strategies. In 2011, Bravewell commissioned a survey on 29 Integrative Medicine Centers and found that 75% reported success using integrative practices to treat chronic pain. More than half of the centers reported positive results for gastrointestinal conditions, depression, anxiety, cancer, and chronic stress.

REFERENCES:

For more information on Maharishi University of Management programs see www.mum.edu.

Dey, S and Pahwa, P, Prakriti and its associations with metabolism, chronic diseases, and genotypes: Possibilities of newborn screening and a lifetime of personalized prevention. *J Ayurveda Integr Med* 2014; 5:15-24

Mahalle, NP et al., Association of constitutional type of Ayurveda with cardiovascular risk factors, inflammatory markers and insulin resistance. *J Ayurveda Integr Med* 2012; 3(3):150-7

Juyal, RC et al., Thelma BK. Potential of ayurgenomics approach in complex trait research: Leads from a pilot study on rheumatoid arthritis. *PLoS ONE* 2012; 7:e45752

Ghodke, Y et al., Traditional Medicine to Modern Pharmacogenomics: Ayurveda Prakriti Type and CYP2C19 Gene Polymorphism Associated with Metabolic Variability. *Evid Based Complement Alternat Med* 2011; 201:249 - 528

Aggarwal, S et al., Indian Genome Variation Consortium. EGLN1 involvement in high-altitude adaptation revealed through genetic analysis of extreme constitution types defined in Ayurveda. *Proc Natl Acad Sci USA* 2010; 107:18961-6

Bhalerao, S et al., Ayurvedic concept of constitution and variations in Platelet aggregation. *BMC Complement Altern Med* 2012; 12:248-56

Tiwari, S et al., Singh G. Effect of walking (aerobic isotonic exercise) on physiological variants with special reference to Prameha (diabetes mellitus) as per Prakriti. *AYU: An International Quarterly Journal of Research in Ayurveda* 2012; 33:44-9

Kurup, RK and Kurup, PA, Hypothalamic digoxin, hemispheric chemical dominance, and the tridosha theory. *Int J Neurosci* 2003; 113(5):657-81·

Tripathi, PK et al., The Basic Cardiovascular responses to postural changes, exercise and cold pressor test: Do they vary in accordance with the dual constitutional types of Ayurveda? *Evid Based Complement Alternat Med* 2011; 201:251-59

Rapolu, SB et al., Physiological variations in the autonomic responses may be related to the constitutional types defined in Ayurveda. *Journal of Humanitas Medicine* 2015; 5(1):e7

Barnes, PM et al., CDC National Health Statistics Report #12. The Use of Complementary and Alternative Medicine in the United States. Findings from the 2007 National Health Interview Survey (NHIS) conducted by the National Center for Complementary and Alternative Medicine (NCCAM) and the National Center for Health Statistics. December 2008

Eisenberg, DM et al., Trends in Alternative Medicine Use in the United States, 1990–1997: Results of a Follow-up National Survey. *JAMA* 1998; 280(18):1569–1575

Ananth, S, Complementary and Alternative Medicine Survey of Hospitals: Summary of Results. Health Forum (American Hospital Association) and the Samueli Institute September 2011. http://www.siib.org/news/2468

For information on Functional Medicine see: https://www.functional-medicine.org/What_is_Functional_Medicine/AboutFM

For information on The Bravewell Collaborative see *www.bravewell.org*

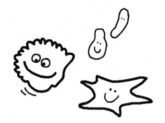

PART 6:

WHAT YOU CAN DO

CHAPTER 32

Dr. Maggie

I recently accompanied a friend to see a gut specialist, Dr. Maggie Ruiz-Paedae. Dr. Maggie is a Doctor of Oriental Medicine, from Florida College of Integrative Medicine, and an expert in Functional Medicine. She radiates enthusiasm and a genuine desire to make her patients healthy. I was especially impressed by her detailed scientific knowledge of the gut. Her treatment program is based on the GAPS diet of Dr. Natasha Campbell-McBride, which we talked about earlier. The diet includes drinking bone broth and taking specific supplements every day. Bone broth is highly valued for healing the gut because it provides nutrients and minerals that culture the beneficial bacteria that can repair a leaky gut. My friend had been a strict vegetarian for years, but because of his health problems, several doctors had recommended that he start to include eggs, fish, and chicken in his diet, so he was prepared to comply with Dr. Maggie's protocol.

The GAPS diet, as we explained, eliminates all grains and many foods that contain sugar. It's recommended that you go on this diet for about a month and then gradually introduce different foods to see how you react. Dr. Maggie makes several exceptions to the GAPS diet. For example, she allows you to have small amounts of coconut palm sugar. She does not recommend probiotics during the first or second phase. It is not until the third phase that the patient begins to use probiotics.

To be on this diet for an extended period, you have to drastically change shopping habits because 80% of the food in most supermarkets contains high fructose corn syrup, one of the worst things you can put in your gut. But it isn't a hard diet for people who enjoy chicken, fish, meat, fruit, veggies, and nuts, with an occasional dairy product. It is similar to the popular Paleo diet.

A huge number of gut doctors (Dr. Axe, Dr. Mercola, Dr. Gundry, Dr. Chutkan, and many others) include different versions of the basic GAPS diet. Dr. Alejandro Junger, for example, uses a version that also eliminates root vegetables, fruit (except berries), coffee, and alcohol, but unlike the other programs, he doesn't recommend bone broth. He also explains in detail how to reintroduce each type of food, and has his own list of supplements, which include probiotics during the first phase.

Whatever differences gut doctors may have, everyone agrees that the first step to health is to repair the gut lining and restore a balanced state of gut bacteria. They all emphasize that a disrupted or leaky gut allows unwanted substances, such as gluten, into the bloodstream, and that these substances are then attacked by our immune system, leading to inflammation. These doctors further agree that sugar is bad for you because it also increases inflammation.

When I asked Dr. Maggie how sugar causes inflammation, she referred me to two YouTube videos (*The Bitter Truth* and *Sugar—An Elephant in the Kitchen*) by Dr. Robert Lustig, a pediatric endocrinologist. Another excellent resource is the bestselling book, *The Case Against Sugar* by Gary Taubes, which, among other things, explains how the sugar industry played a shameful role in misrepresenting fat as the main cause of heart disease and obesity, and portraying sugar as a purely innocent bystander.

I was very interested in several important tests Dr. Maggie recommended for my friend. One of these is a genetic test (HLA typing) used by many doctors to measure two special protein markers on certain immune cells, which help to determine how likely the patient is to have celiac disease. Celiac disease, as you remember, is an intolerance to gluten, and results in damage to the lining of the gut. If you have one of these genetic protein markers for celiac, your chance of having celiac is 1 in 26. If you have both markers, your odds rise to 1 in 7. If you don't have either of these protein markers, you don't have celiac. My friend, for example, was negative for both proteins, and, therefore, will never develop celiac disease. According to Dr. Maggie, the test can also be used to help identify Leaky Gut Syndrome, although this is not an interpretation that would be accepted by most conventional doctors.

She also uses a test that measures lipopolysaccharide (LPS) blood levels. If LPS is high, this suggests the presence of Leaky Gut Syndrome. In addition, the test measures the level of a protein called zonulin, which regulates the tightness of the junction between the cells lining the gut in the small intestine. Knowing the level of zonulin allows the doctor to determine the severity of your condition. This test is also being given by other alternative gut doctors, but is not yet used in conventional medicine.

I was so impressed by Dr. Maggie that I also became her patient. She tried to persuade me to start with only a few tests since they were expensive and many were not covered by insurance, but like a kid in a candy store, I wanted them all. When my friend and I returned for a second visit, we learned that his results were generally good. I, on the other hand, had a more serious situation.

I anxiously awaited my own results, impatiently waiting until Dr. Maggie had finished giving my friend specific recommendations. I glumly assumed that I had a leaky gut and would have to go on a strict diet to heal it. I was shocked to find that, according to Dr. Maggie's analysis, I have had undiagnosed celiac disease for all of my adult life, even though I've experienced only a few symptoms.

Celiac disease can have over 300 different symptoms, so it's no wonder that it takes so long to distinguish it from other conditions. Symptoms can range from mild to extreme. Even testing is complex. The definitive test is a biopsy of the small intestine, but that's often not enough, since other conditions can also cause damage to microvilli. It is also recommended that you have antibody testing as well, but even these results are not conclusive. It's strange that people can have this disease and be completely asymptomatic. You can also be gluten-sensitive without having celiac. The University of Chicago Celiac Disease Center estimates that at least 3 million people are living with celiac disease and

97% of them are undiagnosed. I had never expected to be one of these patients.

Ultimately there's only one treatment for celiac disease—no gluten. And even this isn't clear. Some studies show that people who are gluten-sensitive may also cross-react to other grains, which have gluten-like substances. The good news is that today's patients are more informed, and the Internet has many sites that offer advice and gluten-free recipes.

I'm glad to have Dr. Maggie as my doctor and friend on this challenging journey.

Gut Rap Q & A :

H Bomb: Is this Dr. Maggie qualified to diagnose and treat gut disease?

Doc Gut: She is very well qualified. One of her degrees is a Master's in Medical Technology, and she is more up-to-date on the scientific research than most doctors. She uses state of the art Western diagnostic testing and extensive blood work, combined with dietary and holistic treatments.

Ms. Natural: How did Dr. Maggie discover this path?

Doc Gut: She explains that after getting her degree in medical technology, she worked at a major hospital for six years, mostly with cancer patients and children with AIDS, and then managed a medical facility. Due to continual stress, her health eventually suffered, and she developed depression. She found that the usual medications didn't work for her and she experienced bad side effects. This motivated her to look deeper and find alternatives to conventional medicine.

Ms. Natural: How does she test for SIBO?

Doc Gut: She uses the standard test for SIBO or small intestinal bacteria overgrowth, the same hydrogen breath test used by gastroenterologists.

H Bomb: Does she do any other tests?

Doc Gut: Dr. Maggie does most of the standard blood work normally done by a family physician as well as more advanced tests, depending on her initial analysis of your condition. One very interesting test she does is the MTHFR mutation test. The letters MTHFR stand for methylene tetrahydrofolate reductase, and refer to both an enzyme and the gene that makes the enzyme. It is suggested that as much as half of our population may have MTHFR gene mutations. This can be a problem since the gene plays an important role in many functions, including the metabolism of folic acid and the neutralizing of toxins. Individuals with MTHFR mutations may have an elevated homocysteine level, which is associated with inflammation and an increased risk for heart disease.

H Bomb: Is that test covered by insurance?

Doc Gut: Unfortunately not. Ideally, in the future all these important tests will be.

REFERENCES:

Clean Gut: The Breakthrough Plan for Eliminating the Root Cause of Disease and Revolutionizing Your Health by Dr. Alejandro Junger, HarperOne, Reprint edition 2014

Dr. Lustig, YouTube, *The Bitter Truth*: https://www.youtube.com/watch?v=dBnniua6-oM

Dr. Lustig, YouTube, *Sugar—An Elephant in the Kitchen*: https://www.youtube.com/watch?v=gmC4Rm5cpOI

The Case Against Sugar by Gary Taubes, Knopf, 2016

Kaukinen, K et al., HLA-DQ typing in the diagnosis of celiac disease. *Am J Gastroenterol* 2002; 97(3):695-9.

Sharma, A et al., Identification of Non-HLA Genes Associated with Celiac Disease and Country-Specific Differences in a Large, International Pediatric Cohort. Lee YL, ed. *PLoS ONE* 2016; 11(3):e0152476

Lammi, A et al., Development of gliadin-specific immune responses in children with HLA-associated genetic risk for celiac disease. *Scandinavian Journal of Gastroenterology* 2016; Vol. 51 , Iss. 2,

Moreno-Navarrete, JM et al., Circulating Zonulin, a Marker of Intestinal Permeability, Is Increased in Association with Obesity-Associated Insulin Resistance. Federici M, ed. *PLoS ONE* 2012; 7(5):e37160

University of Chicago Celiac Disease Center fact sheet: https://www.cureceliacdisease.org/wp-content/uploads/341_CDCFactSheets8_FactsFigures.pdf

CHAPTER 33

The Ayurvedic Approach

Ayurveda is particularly suitable for strict vegetarians and others who are not ready to add bone broth to their diet. The majority of the US population knows very little about Ayurveda, but with greater scientific understanding of our gut bacteria, I believe that this situation will change. Western medicine is beginning to learn what Ayurveda has known for millennia—the gut is the key to health.

My experience of Ayurveda came from being with Maharishi Mahesh Yogi as he re-enlivened this ancient science of health. Maharishi spent hundreds of hours with experts from all over India, as well as modern medical doctors and scientists. He worked closely with Dr. Brihaspati Dev Triguna, a master of pulse diagnosis; Dr. Balraj Maharishi, an expert in Dravyaguna, the knowledge of plants and their medical uses, and Dr. V.M. Dwivedi, who possessed the ancient knowledge of rasayanas, in which herbal and mineral preparations are used to prolong life. One of Maharishi's most important contributions was to revitalize specific techniques for the development of consciousness in the practice of Ayurveda. In his honor, this new body of knowledge is referred to as Maharishi Ayurveda.

Two of the simplest and most effective steps Maharishi Ayurveda uses to restore the gut are the elimination of toxins or ama, and the increase of digestive power or agni. Ama, as we explained, includes undigested food or any foreign substance or toxin that gets into the body.

Agni is the digestive power of our gut. It includes the metabolic processes that take place in every tissue of the body. If agni is powerful in these tissues, then our metabolism is powerful and our immune system strong. If our agni is weak, our digestion is weak and ama or toxins leak through the gut wall, accumulating in every tissue, and causing inflammation and disease through-out the body. An Ayurveda physician, or Vaidya, can give you time-tested practical treatment programs to detoxify your body and repair your gut lining.

We briefly reviewed Dr. Kulreet Chaudhary's book *The Prime*, which combines a modern understanding of Integrative Medicine with ancient Ayurveda detox practices. Another recent book on Ayurveda that includes a more traditional Ayurvedic detox and gut repair program is *The Hot Belly Diet* by Dr. Suhas Kshirsagar. Dr. Kshirsagar was trained in Maharishi Ayurveda and, like Dr. Chaudhary, has had a prominent practice in the US. It is useful to go through the details of his program so that we can compare it to the programs of Dr. Maggie and those of other alternative health gut experts.

The main part of *The Hot Belly Diet* is a three-week period in which the patient eats a light diet consisting of a protein shake in the morning, a bowl of *kitchari* (pronounced kit'-cha-ree) at lunch and dinner, and fasts between meals. Kitchari is a liquid soup made from boiled yellow split mung dhal and rice. There are other simple recommendations, such as sipping hot water throughout the day, which also help break down and digest ama.

When our body is not being overwhelmed with food, the ama can be digested more easily and our digestive system has a chance to reboot itself in a process of spontaneous detoxification. In Ayurveda, rekindling agni is called *deepana,* which Dr. Kshirsagar translates as "bioactivator." The elimination of ama is called *pachana,* which he translates as "bioaccelerator."

The programs mentioned in both Dr. Kshirsagar's and Dr. Chaudhary's books are described as weight loss programs, when in fact they include all aspects of health. There are interesting similarities between Dr. Kshirsagar's program and the GAPS diet program used by Dr. Maggie and others. They eliminate hard to digest food, including wheat, dairy, and sugar, for a period of time, and then very gradually reintroduce different foods to determine what it is that is triggering a reaction in your body.

Instead of bone broth, Ayurveda uses kitchari to rest and repair the gut. If a patient's gut lining is too inflamed or damaged to absorb food, Ayurveda will make an exception and it will even prescribe certain animal products for vegetarians or recommend an enema containing a bone broth.

Enemas called *bastis* (bas-tees) are a common practice in Ayurveda. There are different types of bastis with specific purposes. For example, one aims to eliminate toxins while another provides nutrients. The nutritive type of enema or basti consists of specific oils and herbs, and can also contain probiotics in the form of lassi (yogurt taken in the form of a drink consisting of 1 part yogurt to 3 parts water). We can could compare this kind of basti with the probiotic enemas used by alternative medical doctors such as Dr. Perlmutter.

Ayurveda focuses on prevention and includes a number of useful recommendations about how we should eat. One of the easiest and most important tips is that our main meal should always be at lunch. This is because noon is the time when the digestive fires are strongest. Another recommendation is to not have cold or iced drinks with our meals, since cold liquids quench the fire of digestion. Ayurveda also emphasizes eating in a quiet environment so that our attention can be focused on our food, rather than on lively conversation or a TV show. Many people have been helped by Ayurveda treatments, although the number of Western doctors who understand and incorporate these principles into their practices is still small.

One main difference between Ayurveda and alternative health is the emphasis on gluten. Most alternative programs consider gluten to be the cause of gut problems. In Ayurveda, however, wheat is a traditional part of the diet and is generally not excluded.

Dr. John Douillard's book *Eat Wheat: A Scientific and Clinically-Proven Approach to Safely Bringing Wheat and Dairy Back Into Your Diet* refutes many of the claims about the evils of wheat and gluten. Trained in Maharishi Ayurveda, Dr. Douillard explains that wheat has been a natural part of the human diet for much longer than most experts claim. He acknowledges that grains are hard to digest, but suggests that the solution is not the elimination of wheat, but rather the strengthening of our digestive power through Ayurveda. He maintains that processed foods, including gluten-free products, are far worse for us than natural food that contains gluten. I am looking forward to further research to settle this interesting debate.

Gut Rap Q & A:

Ms. Natural: How can we tell if we have excess ama?

Doc Gut: Are your joints stiff? Is your tongue coated in the morning? Do you feel dull and sleepy after eating? Is your mind sometimes foggy? Other symptoms include constipation, diarrhea, lowered immunity, and frequent colds or flu. On the website docgut.com there is a good questionnaire that will help you determine your level of ama.

Ms. Natural: What happens if our ama accumulates over a long period of time?

Doc Gut: It depends on where it settles, and if it blocks any of the fine channels in the body. For example, if ama accumulates in the lungs, the result can be a thick, yellowish toxin, which is fertile ground for bronchial infection. Coronary artery disease is caused by ama blocking the coronary artery.

H Bomb: How do we stop the accumulation?

Doc Gut: As I've mentioned, prevention is key. By changing your diet and lifestyle you can improve digestion and stop the accumulation of ama.

Ms. Natural: What if we slip up on our diet?

Doc Gut: You might be eating a healthy diet and then take a trip and eat the wrong food. One way to correct the situation when you are settled again is to go on an ama-reducing diet for a couple of weeks. This means a lighter diet that includes fresh organic veggies, sweet juicy fruit, whole grains such as quinoa and rice, and easily-digested proteins such as mung dhal or lentil soup.

H Bomb: How do people on an Ayurvedic vegetarian diet get enough protein?

Doc Gut: Vegetarians need to mix foods to get a complete protein. Your food has to have the correct amount of amino acids to be useful to the body. You can ensure this by combining rice and lentils, and including nuts and some milk products every day.

H Bomb: How can ama be equated with toxins, which are generally understood to be poisons?

Doc Gut: It is true that from Western medicine's perspective toxins are specific poisons such as bacteria toxins, chemical waste, or pesticides that are life-threatening and often require you to go immediately to the hospital. In Ayurveda, however, ama doesn't constitute a medical emergency. The toxins are not acutely dangerous, but if they accumulate in the body they will lead to chronic diseases. This is an example of the need to clarify potential misunderstandings and gain a more scientific understanding of the Ayurvedic terms.

Ms. Natural: Is fasting good for everyone?

Doc Gut: No. According to Ayurveda, certain Gut/Brain Natures do not do well fasting, and instead need to have a special light diet designed for them. Any fasting program must be supervised by a trained Ayurveda doctor or Vaidya, based on his analysis of each individual's nature and state of balance.

Ms. Natural: Is there anything else you can do?

Doc Gut: Ayurveda includes an extensive purification program called panchakarma, which has been shown to remove pesticides and other toxins from the body, as well as helping a number of different disorders.

REFERENCES:

Ayurveda: The Science of Self-Healing by Dr. Vasant Lad, Lotus Press, 1985

Maharishi Ayurveda and Vedic Technology: Creating Ideal Health for the Individual and World, Adapted and Updated from The Physiology of Consciousness: Part 2 by Robert Keith Wallace, PhD, Dharma Publications, 2016

The Ageless Woman by Nancy K. Lonsdorf, MD, Maharishi University of Management Press, 2016

The Hot Belly Diet: A 30-day Ayurvedic Plan to Reset your Metabolism, Lose Weight, and Restore Your Body's Natural Balance to Heal Itself by Dr. Suhas Kshirsagar with Kristin Loberg, Atria Books, 2015

Eat Wheat: A Scientific and Clinically-Proven Approach to Safely Bringing Wheat and Dairy Back Into Your Diet by Dr. John Douillard, Morgan James Publishing, 2017

See website at docgut.com for more details on diets. Triphala and other Ayurveda supplements can be obtained from many different sources. We recommend Maharishi Ayurveda Products International (MAPI) because of the purity and high quality of their mostly organic ingredients (see mapi.com).

Herron, RE and Fagan, JB, Lipophil-mediated reduction of toxicants in humans: an evaluation of an ayurvedic detoxification procedure. *Altern Ther Health Med* 2002; 8(5):40-51

For panchakarma treatments see www.theraj.com.

CHAPTER 34

Know Your Gut

One of the big weaknesses of most gut repair programs is their lack of awareness of the individual nature of each person's digestive system. We are all born with different genetic traits and tendencies, so it is not appropriate for each person to have the same diet. Some people might be lactose intolerant, while others may have genes for celiac disease. One person may naturally produce more gas than another, even when they are eating the same food. Some are prone to constipation, others to diarrhea. One individual can skip meals, while another has to eat on time to function well.

Nature and nurture are both important. We know that twins with exactly the same set of genes can have different types of digestion and metabolism. One twin might get fat while the other stays thin. Different genes are turned on in one, but are not active in the other. The genes that are turned on or off at any given time determine the style of functioning of our Gut/Brain network.

We can think of the Gut/Brain network as a computer. The computer hardware is the physical structure of the network and includes the central and peripheral nervous system, enteric nervous system, endocrine system, immune system, and gut bacteria. The computer software is the program that runs that network, which includes the genes that are turned on and the biochemical pathways they control.

The Gut/Brain network processes information in different ways. For example, it can run quickly but with varying degrees of reliability. It can initiate specific routines at preset times and process information in a precise manner. Or it can run in a constant and steady manner, with a high degree of reliability.

We have identified three basic Gut/Brain Natures, which represent both the physical characteristics of the Gut/Brain network and the programs that run it. These three natures are controlled by our individual genetic traits and modified by the particular environment we live in.

The three main Gut/Brain Natures are called:

- Variable Digestive Power or V Gut/Brain

- Pyretic Digestive Power or P Gut/Brain

- Kaloric Digestive Power or K Gut/Brain

The origin of these three basic natures is Ayurveda, and they are called the three main Prakritis. The word Prakriti can be translated as "nature." The Sanskrit words used to describe the three natures are Vata, Pitta, and Kapha. The Variable V Gut/Brain refers to a Vata nature, the Pyretic P Gut refers to a Pitta nature, and the Kaloric K Gut refers to a Kapha nature.

Most systems of natural medicine, for instance, Traditional Chinese Medicine, also use different mind/body types or natures. As we mentioned, recent scientific research using genetic, epigenetic, physiological, and biochemical measures, shows that this ancient individualized approach can be objectively verified. Personalized Medicine uses genetic analysis to help individualize treatments.

Let us take a look at the three gut natures in terms of digestion and mental and emotional behavior. The Variable V Gut/Brain Nature, V Gut for short, refers to people whose digestion tends to be extremely variable, leading to a digestive pattern and appetite that can be strong or weak at different times. These people are "snackers," who enjoy and actually benefit from eating several small nutritious meals throughout the day. When V Gut people become imbalanced, they are prone to constipation and gas and have a sensitive or vulnerable gut that is susceptible to even minor disruptions in their gut bacteria. V Gut people would most likely be prone to irritable bowel syndrome and would benefit from a Low FODMAP Diet. In terms of behavior, they are creative and quick to learn but when out of balance can be unfocused and anxious.

The Pyretic P Gut/Brain Nature represents individuals who have a strong digestive power and appetite. Although the word "pyretic" is defined as feverish, we use it to refer to a reactive fiery gut that produces excess stomach acid. The P Gut individuals need to eat on time. If they don't, they can become irritable and "hangry" (hungry and angry at the same time). We now know that gut bacteria can affect the brain, so perhaps P Gut individuals have a type of gut bacteria whose life cycle requires that they receive food on schedule; otherwise, they might release a chemical that affects certain parts of their brain, which are concerned with the emotion of anger. It would be interesting to decipher the biochemical and neural pathways that are responsible for this "hangry" condition. When these individuals are in a balanced state, their behavior is energetic and purposeful. When out of balance, they can become controlling and aggressive.

The Kaloric or K Gut/Brain person has a slower metabolism and is prone to gaining weight. In Ayurveda, it corresponds to a Kapha nature. Their digestion is stable and they can miss meals without being disturbed. K Gut people enjoy food; however, they must be careful not to overeat. Researchers may eventually show that they have a type of gut bacteria that predisposes them to obesity. These individuals are good-natured and calm when in balance but can become lethargic or depressed when out of balance.

There are also several combinations of these three main natures. (You will find details about each of the Gut/Brain Natures and their possible combinations at docgut.com.) These different Gut/Brain Natures can also be considered in terms of the systems of the body (see first article in the reference section at end of chapter). Interesting research has already identified three basic groups of human gut bacteria called enterotypes (Bacteriodes, Prevotella, and Ruminococcus) and perhaps these can be related to the three main Gut/Brain Natures.

We already know that one of the primary ways to change our gut bacteria and improve our gut health is through diet. By individualizing the diet for each specific Gut/Brain Nature, we can ensure a healthier and more ideal gut bacteria composition.

Gut Rap Q & A

H Bomb: I don't like the idea of being "typed!"

Doc Gut: I understand. No one wants to feel limited, but we all have different characteristics such as blood types, styles of learning, personality traits, etc. Nature has created us as individuals, but we can be grouped by certain shared features. Knowing our individual Gut/Brain Nature allows us to understand specific tendencies and triggers that cause us to go out of balance.

Ms. Natural: What are some other characteristics of each Gut/Brain Nature?

Doc Gut: The Variable V Gut is quite sensitive and benefits greatly from routine. These people are enthusiastic by nature but too much excitement can upset them. Those with a Pyretic P Gut are often good athletes and benefit from strenuous exercise. They like to be in charge and often have strong opinions. Kaloric K Gut people love routines but they need to get off the couch and do something stimulating. They are good friends to all but can become stubborn when out of balance.

You can find more details about your own Gut/Brain Nature, with useful recommendations for staying in balance, by taking the quiz at docgut.com.

Ms. Natural: How do these Gut/Brain Natures compare with the Gut Types described in Dr. Axe's book?

Doc Gut: Dr. Axe's Gut Types are based on Traditional Chinese Medicine. The Gut/Brain Natures we describe in this chapter are based on Ayurveda.

REFERENCES:

Travis, FT, and Wallace, RK, Dosha brain-types: A neural model of individual differences. *J o urnal of Ayurveda and Integral Medicine* 2015; 6, 280-85

Dharma Parenting: Understand your Child's Brilliant Brain for Greater Happiness, Health, Success, and Fulfillment by Robert Keith Wallace, PhD, and Fred Travis, PhD, Tarcher/Perigee, 2016

Maharishi Ayurveda and Vedic Technology: Creating Ideal Health for the Individual and World, Adapted and Updated from The Physiology of Consciousness: Part 2 by Robert Keith Wallace, PhD, Dharma Publications, 2016

See references at the end of Chapter 31 for specific studies on the scien-tific analysis of the main mind/body natures in Ayurveda.

Vernocchi, P et al., Gut Microbiota Profiling: Metabolomics Based Approach to Unravel Compounds Affecting Human Health. *Front Microbiol* 2016; 7:1144

Arumugam, M, et al., Enterotypes of the human gut microbiome. *Nature* 2011, 473,174-180

CHAPTER 35

DHARMA Protocol – Your Roadmap to Health

The Dharma Protocol is your step-by-step method of personal transformation. We recommend it in all our books, which range from parenting to beauty to golf. Dharma is a word with many different meanings. We define dharma as the path in life that brings the greatest happiness, success, and fulfillment.

Dharma Protocol is based on the acronym **D-H-A-R-M-A**:

- **D**iscover: What is your Gut Type or Nature, current gut health, and path for improvement?

- **H**eal: Start a gut health action plan.

- **A**ttention and Appreciation: Stay focused and recognize and appreciate your progress.

- **R**outine: Progressively include lifestyle changes into your routine.

- **M**anage Meltdowns: Damage control and reboot!

- **A**nticipate and Adapt: Prepare for the unexpected and be adaptable.

D stands for Discover

Do you have indigestion, constipation, diarrhea, gas, bloating, acid reflux, or stomach discomfort? If you answer yes to any of these, your gut needs help.

To begin with, decide what approach you want to take to heal your gut. Will you be happier with an alternative practitioner like Dr. Maggie, Dr. Perlmutter, or Dr. Chutkan, or would you like to see an Ayurvedic expert such as Dr. Kshirsagar or Dr. Chaudhary?

All of these approaches will recommend an initial phase of gut detox, rest, and repair, which usually involves a specific diet for several weeks, and eliminates foods that are hard for you to digest. These programs will usually include a nutritious liquid broth or soup to help repair the gut lining. The main difference is that one is designed strictly for meat eaters and one is mainly for vegetarians.

Once your gut has been healed, there are further similarities in treatment between alternative medicine and Ayurveda. For example, Dr. Gundry recommends fasting once a week. This is very Ayurvedic, except that Ayurveda would recommend a different kind of fasting for each Gut/Brain Nature.

Both programs suggest gradually introducing different foods after the initial repair phase in order to determine exactly which foods upset you. Both recommend probiotics. Ayurveda uses probiotics in the form of freshly made food such as yogurt and lassi, while alternative diets also suggest probiotic pills.

Both programs encourage diets that contain fiber when the gut is healed, and both recommend the addition of herbal preparations and supplements. Ayurveda emphasizes traditional herbs and spices, while alternative medicine recommends vitamin, mineral, and other supplements.

The main difference in these approaches is that alternative medicine often recommends one diet for all, while Ayurveda specializes in long-term treatment programs for each individual Gut/ Brain Nature. Ayurveda helps you understand which foods will keep your type in balance, and which foods to avoid. For example, those with a P Gut would be told to avoid hot spices.

How do you choose which approach is best for you? Everyone has their own natural inclination. A meat eater who loves to exercise will almost certainly go for a Paleo diet. A vegetarian and yoga asana practitioner may prefer an Ayurvedic diet. And these aren't the only possible choices. There are many naturopathic doctors, as well as Traditional Chinese Medicine, indigenous healers, energetic healers, and other experts in both modern medicine and natural medicine.

The important thing is to find a doctor or health coach you like and trust. We can't emphasize enough how valuable this is. You need to discover your path and a doctor, health coach, friend, or teacher, to educate and guide you.

H is for Heal Yourself

To heal yourself you must be willing to commit (surrender) to a gut repair program.

A good way to jump-start your program is to do a probiotic enema. You can either follow Dr. Perlmutter's advice or consult an Ayurveda expert (go to docgut.com for useful tips).

Your next step is to make a few simple changes in your lifestyle. This may be as easy as small changes in your diet, exercising regularly, and getting ample sleep. Or it may be more challenging, involving different tests, a strict diet, supplements, probiotics, and prebiotics. Again, a good doctor and mentor makes all the difference. And it's a great help to have a buddy take the journey with you.

We highly recommend starting Transcendental Meditation as a way to reduce stress and rejuvenate your mind and body. It only takes 20 minutes twice a day and will help you make positive changes in every aspect of your life, including digestion.

A is for Attention and Appreciation

Attention or awareness is key to making changes in our lives. It's not easy to give up ingrained habits, and it's better to do it in small steps, with our full attention.

Appreciation and positive support from your friends or family will naturally make your journey to gut health much easier and happier. For example, you could celebrate certain milestones together, which helps them understand how important the process is to you.

R is for Routine

A good way to incorporate new lifestyle changes is to make them part of your daily routine. Whether you're making changes in your diet or adding exercise, you want to integrate them into your schedule so they are as much a part of your life as brushing your teeth.

Everyone approaches routine differently. It's easy for some people, and hard for others. It is good to introduce changes in lifestyle gradually.

M is for Manage Meltdowns

There will be meltdowns, especially if you strain. If your brain is tired or stressed, it's difficult to do anything right. So be aware of the state of your brain and make changes when you are rested.

When you're in the merciless grip of a craving and go off your diet or health program, use Damage Control. Ask yourself, "What is the least harmful thing I can do now to give myself some satisfaction, with the least damage to my gut health?" Then, as soon as possible, reboot your system by restarting your improved routine.

A is for Anticipate and Adapt

Anticipating cravings can help to limit them. For example, don't allow any food into your house that isn't good for you. The less you are tempted, the better! Anticipating means being proactive.

Adapting is essential. If you're at a friend's house and she is serving food that isn't on your list, carefully (and tactfully) avoid the damaging items. If you are traveling, you may not find the food you need, so remember to bring nutritious snacks with you.

ACKNOWLEDGMENTS

We would like to thank
many people who contributed to *Gut Crisis*:
George Foster for his brilliant cover and for formatting
and illustrating the book; Ted and Danielle Wallace
and Gareth Wallace for their feedback and support;
Allen Cobb for his inspiration and creative ideas;
Nicole Windenberger for her excellent editing;
Jim Cody, Toby Leib, Andrew Stenberg, and Joel Silver,
for their thoughtful suggestions; and Fran Clark
for proofreading and copy-editing.

ABOUT THE AUTHORS

ROBERT KEITH WALLACE is a pioneering researcher on the physiology of consciousness. His work has inspired hundreds of studies on the benefits of meditation and other mind-body techniques, and his findings have been published in *Science, American Journal of Physiology,* and *Scientific American.* After receiving his BS in physics and his PhD in physiology from UCLA, he conducted postgraduate research at Harvard University.

Dr. Wallace established the first Maharishi Ayurveda clinics in America, in Fairfield, Iowa; Los Angeles, California; and Washington, DC. He is the director of one of the first master's degree programs in Maharishi Ayurveda and Integrative Medicine in the US.

He serves as Professor and Chairman of the Department of Physiology and Health, Director of Research, and Trustee of Maharishi University of Management (MUM) in Fairfield, Iowa. The author of several books, Dr. Wallace has given hundreds of lectures on Maharishi Consciousness-Based education and health programs around the world.

SAMANTHA WALLACE had a successful career as a model, appearing on the cover of *Vogue* and other magazines and worked with the great photographers of her time, notably Avedon and Penn.

In the summer of 1973, she began to practice Transcendental Meditation.

Devoted to her family and to her practice of meditation, Samantha is a coauthor of *Quantum Golf* with Kjell Enhager, and helps to write and edit her husband's books. She is presently finishing her own book on beauty.

The Wallaces have been happily married for over forty years and have a combined family of four children and six grandchildren.

Index

heart disease ix, xiii, 2, 32, 47, 93, 94, 95, 96, 97, 98, 166, 229, 249, 253
Helicobacter pylori 54, 132, 133
high fructose corn syrup 197, 248
HIV 6, 52, 61
human breast milk 29
human microbiome project 37, 43
hygiene hypothesis 39, 98
hyperlipidemia 6
hypertension 6
hypertriglyceridemia 6

I

IBD vi, 77, 78, 79, 80, 205
IBS 49, 53, 69, 70, 71, 74, 76, 81, 193
Ilya Ilyich Mechnikov xiii
immune cells 46, 47, 77, 78, 87, 95, 100, 108, 109, 110, 114, 195, 249
immune system 16, 29, 39, 46, 64, 84, 86, 87, 94, 100, 108, 114, 116, 117, 166, 201, 228, 248, 256, 266
inflammation ix, 30, 31, 32, 33, 77, 88, 95, 100, 120, 126, 137, 138, 152, 154, 184, 248, 249, 253, 256
inflammatory bowel disease 8, 31, 47, 56, 77, 82, 161, 201, 213
inflammatory response ix, 78, 95, 155
insulin 94, 196, 242
Integrative Medicine 188, 237, 240, 241, 247, 256, 281
irritable bowel syndrome 6, 47, 49, 53, 69, 76, 267

J

Junger, Alejandro 248, 254

K

Kapha 228, 229, 239, 266, 267, 268
ketogenic diet 90
kitchari 257
Kshirsagar, Suhas 256, 263
Kyasanur Forest virus 61

L

L. acidophilus 38, 43, 51
Lactobacillus 9, 16, 51, 52, 54, 70, 85, 86, 200, 201
Lactobacillus plantarum 51, 70, 86

Lactobacillus reuteri 54, 85
Lactobacillus rhamnosus 9, 52
lactose 6, 70, 71, 72, 73, 173, 191, 265
lactose intolerance 6, 191
large intestine 30, 71, 73, 74, 77, 123, 143, 193, 195, 228
Lassa virus 61
lead 22, 57, 58, 86, 94, 95, 96, 100, 166, 180, 261
Leaky Gut Syndrome 119, 120, 121, 124, 227, 249
lectin 125, 165, 166, 169, 170
leprosy 59
leptin 127, 128, 132
lethargy 187
Lifestyle Medicine 237
lipopolysaccharide 152
liver 6, 70, 119, 124, 136, 178, 179, 187, 192
Lyme disease 63

M

Machupo virus 61
Maharishi Ayurveda ii, 141, 184, 235, 237, 256, 259, 263, 272, 281
Maharishi Mahesh Yogi 231, 255
malaria 63, 64, 200, 229
Marburg 61
M cells 111
measles 62
meditation 135, 140, 230, 231, 237, 281
memory 11, 13, 52, 144, 152, 157
Mercola, Joseph 248
Metabolic syndrome 96
metabolomics 49
microbiome xi, 5, 8, 14, 19, 34, 37, 43, 76, 87, 103, 133, 151, 203, 235, 272
Microbiome Medicine 237
microorganisms xi, 29, 37, 38, 39, 41, 46, 51, 65, 136, 138, 197
microvilli 124, 250
minerals 45, 119, 143, 177, 193, 240, 247
monosaccharides 73
motilin 128
MRSA 4, 24, 58, 63
MTHFR 253
mucins 107
mucus 107

multiple sclerosis xiii, 47, 87, 183
Mycobacterium avium paratuberculosis 78
Mycobacterium leprae 59
myelin 87

N

Natasha Campbell-McBride 83, 91, 173, 182, 247
National Institutes of Health xii, 140, 230
Necrotising fasciitis 63
necrotizing enterocolitis 6, 53, 55
nervous system 10, 46, 47, 87, 113, 114, 116, 144, 228, 229, 231, 232, 266
neurological disorders 11, 86, 151, 153, 154, 155
neurotransmitters 47, 114, 116, 130, 231
nutrigenomics 138, 141

O

obesity ix, 1, 2, 3, 5, 8, 16, 19, 26, 27, 30, 31, 32, 34, 93, 96, 97, 128, 130, 132,
    186, 201, 249, 268
odor-sensing receptors 93, 94
ojas 231
oligosaccharides 30, 72
omega-3-essential fatty acid 178
oxalate 201
Oxalobacter formigenes 201

P

Paleo 219, 221, 248, 275
panchakarma 262, 263
Paracatenula 204
Parkinson's xiii, 47, 86, 152, 183
Perlmutter, David 151, 152, 154, 155, 258, 274, 276
Personalized Medicine 237, 267
Peyer's patches 109
Pitta 228, 229, 239, 266, 267
polyols 74
polysaccharide A 87
poop xii, 3, 4, 5, 6, 78, 85, 191, 192, 193, 195
prebiotics 56, 143, 144, 145, 167, 194, 197, 237, 276
Prevotella 39, 268
probiotic enema 153, 154, 276
probiotics ix, xi, xii, xiii, 6, 8, 10, 12, 22, 23, 25, 52, 53, 55, 56, 70, 75, 78, 79,

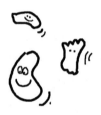

CPSIA information can be obtained
at www.ICGtesting.com
Printed in the USA
BVOW08s0923271017
498822BV00001B/59/P